Healthy You

Easy Weight Loss Guide

Dedication

To all who are on the path to acquiring better health, your courage and dedication are truly inspiring.

To my family and friends, your unwavering support and belief in me have made this possible.

To those who have faced health and weight loss challenges with resilience, your journeys are the heart of this book.

And to everyone striving for a healthier, happier life, this book is dedicated to you. May it serve as your companion and guide you on your journey to wellness.

Acknowledgment

Producing the book "Healthy You" has been an incredible journey, and I could not have done it alone.

First and foremost, I want to thank my family for their unwavering support, encouragement, and love. Your belief in me has been my greatest motivation.

To my friends, thank you for your constant encouragement and for sharing your own health journeys with me. Your insights and experiences have enriched this book in countless ways.

A special thanks to the experts, nutritionists, and fitness professionals who provided invaluable advice and feedback during the writing process. Your knowledge and expertise have helped shape these guides into practical, reliable resources.

To my editor and publishing team, your hard work, patience, and dedication have been instrumental in bringing this book to life. Thank you for believing in this project and for your meticulous attention to detail.

Lastly, to all the readers, thank you for choosing this book as part of your health and wellness journey. Your commitment to improving your health is truly inspiring. I hope this guide helps you achieve your goals and lead a healthier, happier life.

With gratitude, Alona Rose Goldman

About the Author

Born in Belarus, Alona Rose Goldman is a 38-year-old dedicated health and wellness enthusiast with a passion for helping others achieve their best selves. She migrated to the United States 12 years ago and is now a US Citizen living in Miami, Florida. With years of experience in the field of nutrition, fitness, and holistic health, Goldman has guided countless individuals on their journeys to achieve better health and well-being.

Holding a degree in Nutrition Science, she combines professional expertise with personal experience to provide practical, effective strategies for weight loss and overall wellness. She believes that a balanced approach to health is the key to sustainable results and lasting happiness.

In "Healthy You," Goldman shares her comprehensive knowledge in an accessible and motivating way, empowering readers to take control of their health and transform their lives. She is committed to making healthy living achievable and enjoyable for everyone.

When not writing or coaching, she enjoys cooking healthy meals, hiking, weight lifting, swimming, practicing yoga, and spending time with her family and friends.

Goldman is a passionate advocate for holistic health and longevity, dedicated to helping others achieve a balanced and fulfilling life. With a background in Nutrition Science, she has spent 18 years researching and implementing effective strategies for optimal health and wellness.

Alona Goldman's approach is rooted in the belief that living a long and healthy life is attainable through a combination of proper nutrition, regular physical activity, mental well-being, and positive lifestyle choices. She has helped countless individuals transform their lives through personalized health plans and one-on-one coaching.

In "Healthy You," Goldman distills her extensive knowledge into practical advice and actionable steps, making it easy for readers to incorporate healthy habits into their daily routines. With a focus on sustainability and enjoyment, she aims to inspire and empower readers to take charge of their health for the long term.

Preface

Welcome to "Healthy You," a journey into the heart of personalized nutrition and sustainable weight loss. In a world where fad diets and quick fixes are tantalizingly advertised on every corner, this book is a beacon for those who seek a more profound and lasting transformation. It's about more than just shedding pounds; it's about reclaiming your vitality, embracing a balanced lifestyle, and nurturing a relationship with food that enhances every aspect of your life.

The idea for "Healthy You" was born out of a simple yet powerful observation: every individual is unique, and so, too, should be their approach to health and wellness. We are not one-size-fits-all, and our diets shouldn't be either. Through years of research, experience, and listening to countless stories of triumph and struggle, it became clear that the most successful and sustainable weight loss journeys are those tailored to the individual, taking into account their lifestyle, preferences, and goals.

This book is not a prescriptive diet manual, nor does it promise overnight results. Instead, it offers a roadmap to understanding your body's needs and developing a personalized plan that you can maintain for life. We'll go into the science of nutrition, the psychology of eating, and the practicalities of planning and preparing meals that nourish both body and soul. You'll find tools and strategies to help you overcome obstacles, stay motivated, and celebrate your progress.

"Healthy You" is divided into comprehensive sections, each designed to guide you step-by-step through the process of creating your personalized diet plan. From assessing your current eating habits to setting realistic goals, from understanding the role of macronutrients to learning how to listen to your body's hunger cues, every chapter is crafted to empower you with knowledge and confidence.

As you begin this book, remember that the path to a healthier you is not a straight line but a series of steps, each one bringing you closer to your goals. There will be challenges and setbacks, but there will also be victories and moments of profound self-discovery. This book is your companion and guide, here to support you every step of the way.

To everyone who has ever struggled with their weight, felt overwhelmed by dietary choices, or doubted their ability to make lasting changes – this book is for you. May "Healthy You" inspire you to take control of your health, embrace the power of personalized nutrition, and discover the best version of yourself.

Here's to your journey toward a healthier, happier you.

With warmest regards,

Alona

Contents

Chapter 1: Setting the Foundation for Sustainable Weight Loss

Starting a sustainable weight loss plan requires setting a solid foundation like that of a durable building that withstands the test of time. This chapter explores the critical elements of creating a powerful base for your weight loss journey. I will walk you through my personal journey, help you understand the science behind sustainable weight loss, and encourage you to integrate a holistic strategy into your lifestyle.

My Personal Journey as an Integrative Nutritionist and Health Coach

In this section, I'm excited to share with you the story of my own transformation, which propelled me into a career as an integrative nutritionist and health coach. My journey toward embracing sustainable weight loss and enhancing my overall health began out of a personal struggle. Like many, I was once overly concerned with my weight and outward appearance, caught in a cycle of fad diets and intensive exercise regimes that offered only temporary solutions.

It wasn't until I stumbled upon the principles of integrative nutrition that a new horizon opened up for me. This was not just another diet trend but a holistic approach to health that finally felt balanced and sustainable. The deeper I delved into nutrition and health sciences, the clearer it became that weight loss isn't a one-size-fits-all affair. Our individuality, encompassing our dietary needs, lifestyle habits, and personal health goals, plays a crucial role in shaping our approach to losing weight.

Motivated by these insights, I pursued and achieved certification as an integrative nutritionist and health coach. This journey wasn't just for my own benefit; it was fueled by a desire to guide others through the often-confusing world of diet and health, helping them find their own path to success.

Working closely with clients, I've witnessed the incredible changes a personalized diet plan can bring. By acknowledging and respecting each person's unique needs and tastes, I've helped many achieve not just temporary weight loss but lasting health improvements.

My experiences have taught me an invaluable lesson: sustainable weight loss transcends mere calorie counting and strict dieting. It's about discovering a lifestyle balance that nourishes both the body and mind. By focusing on whole, nutrient-rich foods, adopting mindful eating habits, and making positive lifestyle adjustments, achieving your weight loss goals and enhancing your health is entirely possible.

I share my journey with the hope that it will encourage you to take the reins of your own health and explore a weight loss path tailored just for you. With dedicated guidance and support, I believe anyone can reach their wellness goals and lead a more fulfilling, healthier life.

A Holistic Approach to Weight Loss for Long-Term Success

Achieving lasting weight loss goes far beyond the simplistic formula of dieting; it necessitates a comprehensive approach that encompasses every facet of your health and daily life. This holistic strategy extends its focus beyond mere dietary habits to include crucial elements like stress management, sleep quality, physical activity, and hydration—all of which significantly influence your journey toward a healthier weight.

Central to this holistic viewpoint is the concept of personalized diet plans. Recognizing that every individual has distinct nutritional requirements, tastes, and objectives underscores the importance of tailoring diet plans. A diet that aligns with your unique lifestyle and preferences is not only more enjoyable but also sustainable in the long run.

But there's more to it than just what you eat. Regular physical activity, effective stress management techniques, prioritizing restful sleep, and staying well-hydrated are essential components of a successful weight loss strategy. Each of these factors contributes significantly to your overall well-being and plays a critical role in your ability to lose weight sustainably.

Moreover, a holistic approach to weight loss also means paying attention to your mental and emotional health. It's common to find solace in food during times of stress, anxiety, or emotional upheaval. Addressing these underlying emotional triggers and discovering healthier coping mechanisms can help you overcome patterns of emotional eating, paving the way for true and lasting weight loss success.

Hence, a holistic approach to losing weight involves a comprehensive consideration of your overall health and lifestyle. By crafting a diet plan that's uniquely yours, engaging in regular physical activity, managing stress, ensuring quality sleep, and addressing emotional well-being, you're setting the stage for long-term success on your weight loss journey.

The Science Behind Sustainable Weight Loss

Achieving sustainable weight loss requires a solid grasp of the science that underpins it. This journey extends beyond the temporary allure of fad diets or the fleeting commitment to rigorous exercise regimes. The essence of sustainable weight loss lies in adopting lifestyle modifications that you can maintain over the long haul, ensuring a healthy weight for years to come.

At the heart of sustainable weight loss is the principle of creating a calorie deficit—burning more calories than you consume. However, this needs to be approached in a healthy and sustainable manner. Extreme diets that drastically cut calories can be detrimental, leading to nutrient deficiencies and other health issues.

Understanding the significance of macronutrients—carbohydrates, proteins, and fats—is another pivotal aspect. These are the building blocks of your diet and play crucial roles in energy balance and metabolism. By learning how to properly balance these nutrients, you can enhance your weight loss efforts and bolster your health.

Physical activity is equally essential. Regular exercise does more than just burn calories; it also promotes cardiovascular health, elevates your mood, and helps alleviate stress. A balanced approach, incorporating both dietary changes and physical activity, is key to maximizing your weight loss success and boosting your overall health.

In essence, sustainable weight loss is about more than just shedding pounds; it's about making informed, lasting changes to your eating habits and lifestyle. By delving into the science of weight loss and making educated decisions about your diet and activity levels, you can achieve enduring success and maintain a healthy weight throughout your life.

Chapter 2: Embracing Your Uniqueness

In the world of weight loss and health, recognizing and celebrating our individuality is paramount. In this chapter, you'll learn how we are all beautifully distinct, with diverse bodies, metabolisms, and nutritional needs. You'll discover what uniquely works for you in the realm of sustainable weight loss and overall health.

So, let's embrace the journey of understanding and catering to your body's specific needs, as this is the cornerstone of not just achieving but also maintaining optimal health and weight.

Genetics and Metabolism

When embarking on a weight loss journey, understanding the interplay between genetics, metabolism, and body type is essential. These factors significantly influence how our bodies process foods, store fats, and respond to physical activities. Tailoring your diet and exercise plan according to your unique genetic profile, metabolic rate, and body shape can enhance your efforts toward sustainable weight loss, ensuring you achieve and maintain your goals in the long run.

Genetics is a key player in shaping our body types and how we metabolize different nutrients, impacting our responses to various diets and exercise routines. For instance, some individuals might find themselves predisposed to accumulate fat more readily due to their genetic makeup, whereas others might enjoy a naturally higher metabolic rate, allowing them to burn calories faster.

Recent research has increasingly highlighted the significant role that genetics plays in determining our body composition, how we metabolize nutrients, and our individual responses to different diets and exercise routines. A study published on PubMed discusses the genetic aspects of body composition, emphasizing that traits such as fat distribution and muscle mass have high heritability estimates ranging from 0.4 to 0.7. This suggests that genetics significantly influences these traits. Moreover, the study highlights the identification of major genes controlling products like leptin, which play crucial roles in appetite and energy expenditure control, thereby affecting body composition[1].

Nutrigenomics is a field that explores the relationship between nutrition and the genome. It posits that genetic variations can affect how individuals metabolize nutrients, which in turn influences dietary requirements and responses to certain diets. References from the NCBI Bookshelf elaborate on the concept of nutrigenomics, indicating that genetic predispositions can inform dietary recommendations and interventions tailored to individual genetic profiles[2]. This personalized approach to nutrition underscores the importance of genetics in dietary metabolism and its potential to optimize health outcomes.

---

[1] https://pubmed.ncbi.nlm.nih.gov/10422098/
[2] https://www.ncbi.nlm.nih.gov/books/NBK518614/

By gaining insights into your genetic tendencies, you can make more informed decisions regarding the foods and workouts that will most effectively support your weight loss journey.

Adopting a diet that aligns with your genetic makeup involves understanding how your genes influence your reaction to certain nutrients and your overall dietary habits. Although genetic testing can shed light on your predispositions, it's important to remember that genetics is just one of many factors affecting your nutritional requirements and how you respond to specific diets. Here are steps to leverage genetic information for tailoring your diet:

Step 1: Consult with a Professional: Engage with a healthcare provider, such as a registered dietitian or a genetic counselor, who can help interpret your genetic test results.

Step 2: Understand Genetic Impacts: Discuss how certain genetic variations may affect your needs for nutrients, your food preferences, and your body's tolerance to specific foods.

Step 3: Identify Metabolic Traits: Pay attention to genetic markers that influence your metabolism of key macronutrients like carbohydrates, fats, and proteins.

Step 4: Personalize Your Diet: Utilize the insights obtained from your genetic profile to customize your diet, ensuring it meets your individual requirements.

Step 5: Adjust Macronutrient Balance: Modify the ratios of carbohydrates, fats, and proteins in your diet based on your genetic predispositions and metabolic characteristics.

Moreover, metabolism plays a pivotal role in your weight loss journey. It refers to the biochemical processes that occur within a human body to maintain life, including the conversion of food and drink into energy. This energy is essential for various bodily functions, such as breathing, circulating blood, and cell repair. The efficiency and speed of these metabolic processes can influence an individual's ability to lose weight, making metabolism a pivotal factor in the weight loss journey.

It's important to understand here that when calories are restricted for weight loss, the body adapts by slowing down the metabolic rate to conserve energy, a phenomenon known as metabolic adaptation. This adaptation can make continued weight loss challenging and is a key factor in the common experience of weight loss plateaus.

Equally critical is the fact that exercise is a significant metabolism booster. Physical activity helps build lean muscle mass, which is more metabolically active than fat tissue. This means that individuals with a higher proportion of muscle mass have a higher BMR and burn more calories at rest. Regular exercise, therefore, not only contributes directly to calorie expenditure but also indirectly supports weight loss by enhancing metabolic rate[3].

Therefore, understanding and adapting your diet plan to your metabolic rate is essential for achieving your weight loss or maintenance goals effectively.

---

[3] https://www.ncbi.nlm.nih.gov/books/NBK572145/

Here are detailed steps to customize your diet based on your metabolism:

Step 1: Calculate Your Basal Metabolic Rate (BMR)

Begin by determining your BMR, which is the amount of energy (in calories) your body requires to perform basic life-sustaining functions at rest. You can use online BMR calculators that factor in your age, gender, weight, height, and activity level to estimate your daily caloric needs.

Step 2: Adjust Your Caloric Intake

With your BMR in mind, tailor your daily calorie consumption to align with your weight loss objectives. To maintain your current weight, your calorie intake should match your BMR. For weight loss, consume fewer calories than your BMR to create a caloric deficit. Conversely, to gain weight, your intake should exceed your BMR.

Step 3: Customize Macronutrient Ratios

Tailor your intake of macronutrients—carbohydrates, proteins, and fats—according to your metabolic profile and personal goals. Those with faster metabolisms or who are more active might require more carbohydrates for energy. Meanwhile, individuals with slower metabolisms or insulin sensitivity may benefit from reducing carbohydrate intake in favor of increasing protein and healthy fats to enhance satiety and support muscle maintenance.

Step 4: Focus on Nutrient-Dense Foods

Independent of your metabolic rate, prioritize the consumption of nutrient-rich foods, such as fruits, vegetables, whole grains, lean proteins, and healthy fats. Always start your meal with a big bowl of salad and vegetables because they are high in fiber and low in calories. Vegetables are also high-volume, low-calorie foods. They contain fiber and water, which add bulk to your meals and help fill you up. High-fiber foods not only provide volume but also take longer to digest, making you feel full on fewer calories for longer periods. Choose high-quality, minimally processed items that offer vital nutrients like vitamins, minerals, fiber, and antioxidants that boost overall health and metabolic function.

Step 5: Experiment with Meal Timing and Frequency

Metabolic response to the timing and frequency of meals varies among individuals. Some may find that eating smaller, more frequent meals throughout the day helps maintain an active metabolism. Others might prefer fewer, larger meals. Test different eating schedules to see how your body reacts regarding energy, hunger, and fullness.

Step 6: Monitor and Adjust

Keep a close eye on your progress, adjusting your dietary plan as necessary based on changes in your weight, energy levels, and overall sense of well-being. Stay patient and flexible; metabolic rates can change due to various factors, including aging, hormonal shifts, activity levels, and changes in eating habits.

Understanding and tailoring your approach to diet and exercise based on your genetics and metabolism can significantly enhance your path to sustainable weight loss. Recognizing the uniqueness of each individual is key; what effectively aids one person in their weight loss journey might not yield the same results for another. By gaining insight into your own body's specific needs and preferences and making informed, personalized choices accordingly, you're more likely to find a sustainable and successful path to weight management. This bespoke approach ensures that your diet and exercise plan not only supports weight loss but also nurtures your overall health and well-being, paving the way for long-term success and a healthier lifestyle.

Hormonal Balance

Achieving sustainable weight loss significantly hinges on the hormonal balance within our bodies. A diet mindful of hormonal influences involves a deep understanding of how hormones like insulin, cortisol, and leptin affect metabolism, appetite, energy levels, and overall health. Hormonal imbalances can lead to challenges in managing weight, as they may cause increased fat storage and appetite, making weight loss more difficult.

Consulting with a healthcare professional, particularly an endocrinologist, to evaluate your hormone levels through blood tests is a strategic step. This evaluation can uncover any imbalances, paving the way for a tailored diet plan that addresses these specific issues.

Insulin, a hormone crucial for blood sugar regulation, can lead to weight gain when levels spike due to excessive intake of refined carbohydrates and sugars. A diet emphasizing whole foods, lean proteins, and healthy fats can help maintain stable insulin levels, facilitating weight loss.

Cortisol, known as the stress hormone, influences weight by increasing appetite and encouraging fat storage, particularly in the abdominal area, under chronic stress conditions. Integrating stress-reduction practices such as yoga, meditation, and consistent physical activity into your routine can help mitigate cortisol's impact, aiding in weight loss.

Leptin, responsible for regulating hunger and energy usage, can lead to heightened hunger and overeating when out of balance. A diet abundant in fiber, protein, and healthy fats can enhance leptin sensitivity and support feelings of fullness, aiding in weight management.

Adopting lifestyle modifications that encourage hormonal equilibrium, including regular physical activity, effective stress management, and a diet rich in balanced nutrients, is key to promoting long-term weight loss. By recognizing the profound influence of hormones on weight and general health, we can develop a personalized dietary and lifestyle blueprint that fosters long-term success and enhanced well-being.

Chapter 3: Setting Your Goals

Establishing health and wellness goals is a foundational step towards attaining sustainable weight loss and enhancing your overall well-being. These goals act as guiding lights, providing both direction and motivation as you navigate through your journey of self-improvement. In this chapter, we delve into the significance of setting concrete objectives and how they can shape your path to a healthier you.

Importance of Health and Wellness Goals

Having clear health and wellness goals sets the stage for a focused approach to weight loss and health enhancement. It allows you to customize your dietary habits and exercise routines in alignment with your aspirations. Whether you're aiming to shed pounds, boost your physical fitness, or simply lead a healthier life, setting explicit goals helps in devising a plan that's specifically catered to those ambitions. This targeted strategy not only aids in tracking your progress but also ensures that you're making adjustments that genuinely contribute to your overarching aims.

Moreover, goals act as a relentless source of motivation. The journey towards weight loss and better health is often long and filled with challenges. However, having a clear endpoint in sight can significantly bolster your dedication and perseverance. Celebrating each milestone achieved along the way not only reinforces your confidence but also reinvigorates your commitment to continue striving forward.

Beyond serving as a motivational tool, setting specific health and wellness objectives empowers you to make educated decisions regarding your nutrition and lifestyle. It encourages a deep dive into your habits, helping you pinpoint areas that need refinement. Armed with this insight, you can craft a personalized action plan that not only suits your unique preferences but also effectively addresses your individual health needs, thereby elevating your chances of achieving enduring success and maintaining a healthy lifestyle over the long term.

In essence, health and wellness goals are not just milestones to be reached; they are the very framework upon which sustainable weight loss and a vibrant, healthy life are built. By embracing the process of setting and pursuing these goals, you lay down the groundwork for a personalized, informed, and ultimately successful journey toward lasting well-being.

SMART Goals Technique

In any endeavor towards losing weight and improving health, the act of goal-setting is pivotal. However, employing the SMART goals technique elevates this process, transforming aspirations into tangible, attainable objectives. This methodical approach breaks down goals into five critical attributes: Specific, Measurable, Achievable, Relevant, and Time-bound, making the journey towards sustainable weight loss more structured and achievable.

Specific: Clarity is key. Define your goal with precision to give your weight loss journey a clear direction. For example, rather than a vague "I want to lose weight, " opt for a defined target like, "I aim to lose 10 pounds within the next three months." This specificity provides a solid target to aim for.

Measurable: To gauge your progress, your goal must be quantifiable. This could mean weekly weigh-ins to monitor weight loss or using a tape measure to track changes in body measurements. Measuring progress not only shows how far you've come but also keeps you motivated to continue.

Achievable: While ambition is important, realism is crucial. Set goals that challenge you without setting the bar too high. Begin with smaller, manageable goals, gradually escalating your targets as you build confidence and capability. This approach helps maintain momentum and prevents discouragement.

Relevant: Ensure your goals align with your broader health aspirations and personal values. A goal that resonates with you on a personal level will be more motivating and meaningful, driving you to persist even when faced with obstacles.

Time-bound: Incorporating a deadline into your goal instills a sense of urgency and focus. Without a specified timeframe, it's easy to defer efforts and lose sight of your objectives. Establish a practical deadline to achieve your goal, promoting a steady pace towards your target.

SMART goals are beneficial for several reasons. They provide clarity by helping individuals identify exactly what they want to achieve and monitor their progress. They are also motivational, as setting achievable goals can keep individuals motivated and on track during their recovery process. Additionally, SMART goals foster self-empowerment by allowing individuals to take charge of their recovery and increase their confidence in their ability to overcome obstacles. Lastly, sharing goals with others and having a support system in place can increase accountability and motivation[4].

Thus, adopting the SMART goals framework offers a pragmatic roadmap to navigate your weight loss journey, enhancing the likelihood of enduring success. It's also important to periodically review and adjust your goals as necessary, ensuring they remain aligned with your evolving needs and circumstances. By setting and pursuing SMART goals, you're not just aspiring to lose weight; you're methodically working towards a healthier, more fulfilling life.

Prioritizing and Celebrating Milestones

On the path to sustainable weight loss, recognizing and rejoicing in milestones is crucial. These markers of progress encompass much more than merely observing numerical changes on the scale; they celebrate the smaller yet significant victories that collectively contribute to lasting success. Acknowledging these moments of achievement keeps you driven and dedicated to your objectives.

Achieving small goals along the way can provide a sense of accomplishment and reinforce the idea that progress is possible[5]. Reflecting on these achievements can also serve as a reminder of the individual's commitment to their health and wellness goals, further motivating them to continue their efforts.

---

[4] https://www.aquilarecoveryva.com/blog/setting-smart-goals-recovery
[5] https://www.bhf.org.uk/informationsupport/heart-matters-magazine/wellbeing/how-to-motivate-yourself-to-get-healthy

Celebrating these milestones as you reach them is equally important. Celebrations could be as modest as enjoying a favorite healthy dish or as rewarding as purchasing new fitness attire. These acts of celebration not only reward your hard work but also bolster a sense of achievement, reinforcing the positive steps you've taken and energizing your continued journey toward health and weight loss.

In summary, goal-setting is a crucial step in reviving your health, but to have a real impact, your goals need to be SMART. On top of that, you must reward yourself along the way for every milestone you accomplish. In the next chapter, we'll take a deep dive into the power of nutrition in assisting you achieve your health and wellness goals.

Chapter 4: Nutrition: Nourishing Your Body

Eating right is the most important part of losing weight and keeping it off. Learning about healthy eating helps you make smart food choices. This helps you lose weight and makes you healthier and happier. This part of the book teaches you the simple facts and steps you need to know about what you eat and how it helps you.

Fundamentals of Nutrition

It's important to understand here that food nutrients are broadly categorized into two types: macronutrients and micronutrients.

Macronutrients are further classified into three main types, namely carbohydrates, proteins, and fats. Your body needs these nutrients to gain energy and function properly. Knowing about these nutrients helps you pick the right foods for your meals. This way, you can eat in a way that not only helps you lose weight but also lets you stay healthy overall. Here are some basic details on how these nutrients can be attained:

- Carbohydrates are found in foods like whole grains: brown rice, quinoa, millet, legumes, starchy vegetables. They give you the energy to stay active.

- Proteins come from meat, fish, and legumes. They help build and repair your muscles as well as other parts of your body.

- Fats like avocado and olive oils, lean meat like turkey or chicken fillet, fatty fish like salmon and cod, avocado, and raw nuts. Fats are essential for optimizing your health and helping you stay energetic.

Besides the macronutrients, we also need to pay attention to vitamins and minerals. These are micronutrients.

Micronutrients are vitamins and minerals required by the body for many processes, growth, and functioning. They are found in every food group, including fruits, vegetables, whole grains, lean proteins, and fats. Eating a variety of foods each day is the best way to get all the micronutrients you need.

Besides, micronutrients are required for optimal nutrition, to boost immune function, to support many body structures and processes, and to help protect against diseases and other health conditions.

They help keep our bones strong, heal cuts, fight off germs, and give us energy. Some important micronutrients include vitamins A, C, D, E, K, and B, and minerals like calcium for strong bones, iron for healthy blood, magnesium for muscles, and zinc to help fight off sickness.

Another important part of eating right is knowing how much to eat. This means listening to your body and eating only when you're really hungry, not just because you're bored or because the food tastes good. This can help you avoid overeating and lose weight slowly and in a healthy way.

Hence, staying healthy is all about making smart choices about what you eat and how much you eat. Let's take a look at some dietary approaches to make this possible:

Dietary Approaches: Mindful and Balanced Eating

One big part of ensuring optimal health and shedding some pounds is learning to eat mindfully and in a balanced way. This means really paying attention to what you eat and choosing foods that are good for your health and well-being. When you eat mindfully, you focus on your food. You notice how it tastes, how it smells, and even how you feel when you eat it.

Eating mindfully helps you enjoy your food more. It's about enjoying what you eat without making unhealthy food choices.

Studies have found that mindful eating can be really good for your health. For example, it can help lower unhealthy fats in your blood and increase good fats, which lowers your chance of getting heart disease. It might also help maintain your blood sugar because you might eat less sugary foods. Eating this way can even help you improve gut health[6].

Balanced eating is about making sure your meals have lots of different healthy foods. This includes eating vegetables, fruits, whole grains (like brown rice, quinoa, legumes, millet, buckwheat), lean proteins (foods that give you good muscle-building material like chicken or beans), and healthy fats (like olive oil or nuts). Eating a variety of these foods makes sure your body gets all the different nutrients it needs to work really well.

It's important to understand that there's no single route to staying healthy. It works differently for everyone. What works well for one person might not work for someone else. Knowing this helps you figure out the best way to eat right for your own

---

[6] https://www.usnews.com/wellness/food/articles/benefits-of-mindful-eating

body type. You can choose foods you like and those that are good for you, making your diet something you enjoy and can stick with for a long time.

Here are some easy tips for eating mindfully and in a balanced way every day:

- Eat slowly and enjoy each bite. This helps you enjoy your food more and know when you're full.

- Listen to your body. Eat when you're hungry and stop when you're full.

- Plan what you're going to eat ahead of time. Make sure your meals have a good mix of nutrients.

- Watch how much you eat. Make sure you're eating enough for your body, but not too much.

- Try to eat different foods. This makes sure you get all kinds of nutrients and keeps meals fun.

Adding these habits to your daily routine can help you lose weight in a good way. You'll enjoy your food more and feel better. This approach is key to losing weight while optimizing your overall well-being.

Nutrition Plan

Eating the right foods is very important for losing weight the right way. Making a good plan for what to eat can help you reach and keep up with your weight goals.

A good food plan is more than just counting calories or not eating certain kinds of food. It's about making sure you eat the right kinds of food that give your body the energy and nutrients it needs for your everyday life and for losing weight. It's important to make a plan that fits your own likes, what you need, and your goals. This way, you can stick with it, and it will work better for you.

When creating a good food plan, it is essential to choose whole foods that are full of nutrients. These foods are really important for a healthy diet because they have lots of vitamins and minerals that help your body maintain its optimal functioning. As discussed earlier, eating a mix of vegetables, fruits, whole grains (like oats, brown rice, quinoa, buckwheat, legumes), lean proteins (like chicken, fish or turkey), and healthy fats (like avocados and nuts) is what you need. This kind of eating gives you more energy and enhances your overall health.

Drinking enough water and choosing your drinks wisely is also very important. When it comes to our health, it's clear that sugary drinks should be avoided. Water and unsweetened herbal teas are a great choice because they keep you hydrated without adding any extra calories that your body doesn't need.

Fad Diets

Many people are drawn to quick-fix diets that promise fast weight loss. These diets often tell you to eat a lot of a single kind of food or to not eat certain types of food at all. While they might make you lose weight quickly at first, these diets don't usually work well in the long run and can even be detrimental to your health.

When you don't eat certain foods or cut calories too much, you might not get all the nutrients your body needs. This can make you lose muscle, not just fat, and can increase your chance of heart disease. Also, these diets can lead to losing and then gaining weight over and over again, a cycle known as yo-yo dieting. This is not good for your health and can lead to serious problems like eating disorders, not getting enough nutrients, feeling unhappy, weak bones, not enough iron in your blood, problems with your body's metabolism, hormonal deficiencies, and heart issues[7].

One big problem with quick-fix diets is that they're the same for everyone. But since everyone's body, way of life, and goals are different, a one-size-fits-all diet doesn't work well for everybody. Finding the right way to maintain good health is a personal journey. You need a plan that's made just for you, taking into account what you need and like.

Our goal should thus be to choose diet plans that really work for a long time, not just quick fixes that don't last.

Importance of Whole Food Plant-Based Diet

Plant-based or plant-forward eating patterns focus on foods that come primarily from plants. These include not only fruits and vegetables but also nuts, seeds, oils, whole grains, legumes, and beans. Choosing these items doesn't make you a vegetarian or vegan, nor do they mean that you never eat meat or dairy. Rather, it's just that you are proportionately choosing more of

---

[7] https://extension.okstate.edu/fact-sheets/the-health-risk-of-fad-diets.html

your foods from plant sources than other food groups. Eating a diet based on whole plant foods is a highly effective way to lose weight and get healthier. This kind of diet means eating foods like vegetables, fruits, whole grains, nuts, seeds, and beans. These foods are close to their natural state and not heavily processed. This way of eating focuses on the variety and benefits of eating plants.

Choosing unprocessed plant-based foods helps you cut down on unhealthy sugars and fats without counting every calorie. You can still feel full and satisfied because these foods are good for you. This makes losing weight easier and more natural, helping you have a healthier way of eating without feeling restricted.

A diet rich in whole plant-based foods is full of nutrients that are good for you. It has lots of vitamins, minerals, and fibers, which help your body in many ways. The antioxidants in these foods can reduce inflammation and lower your risk of diseases like heart disease and diabetes. Fiber helps your digestion, keeps your blood sugar steady, and helps keep your cholesterol in a healthy range. All these benefits help improve your overall health, making your body work better.

Switching to a diet full of whole, plant-based foods helps you lose weight and makes your whole body healthier. This kind of diet can lower your chances of getting long-term health problems like heart disease, type 2 diabetes, and some kinds of cancer. In fact, this dietary approach isn't just good for you; it's also good for our planet. A whole plant-based diet uses fewer resources and causes less harm to the environment, so it's an environment-friendly choice.

A whole-foods, plant-based shopping list

Fruits: Berries, citrus fruits, pears, peaches, pineapple, bananas, etc.

Vegetables: Kale, spinach, tomatoes, broccoli, cauliflower, asparagus, peppers, etc.

Starchy vegetables: Sweet potatoes, butternut squash, carrots, beets, etc.

Whole grains: oats, farro, quinoa, brown rice pasta, barley, etc.

Healthy fats: Avocados, nuts, and olive oil.

Legumes: Peas, chickpeas, lentils, nuts, beans, etc.

Seeds, nuts, and nut butters: Almonds, cashews, macadamia nuts, pumpkin seeds, sunflower seeds, tahini, brazil nuts, etc.

Unsweetened plant-based milks: Almond milk, macadamia nut milk, etc.

Spices, herbs, and seasonings: Basil, rosemary, turmeric, curry, black pepper, ginger, etc.

Condiments: Mustard, nutritional yeast, apple cider vinegar, lemon juice, etc.

Plant-based protein: soybeans, low sodium tofu and tempeh or plant based protein powders with no added sugar or artificial ingredients.

Beverages: Unsweetened coffee or tea, spring water, etc.

When supplementing your plant-based diet with animal products, choose high-quality products from grocery stores or, better yet, purchase them from local farms. Examples of animal products that can be enjoyed in moderation include:

- Eggs (egg yolk is high in cholesterol)

- poultry

- beef

- low-fat dairy products

While you can consume conventional animal products, some people may choose pasture-raised, grass-fed, wild-caught, or organic products for environmental reasons or personal preferences.

A healthy WFPB diet should focus on plant foods like vegetables, fruits, whole grains, legumes, nuts, and seeds. If animal products are eaten, they should be eaten in smaller quantities compared to plant foods.

The WFPB diet is a way of eating that focuses on consuming foods in their most natural form. This means that heavily processed foods are excluded.

When purchasing groceries, focus on fresh foods, and when purchasing foods with a label, aim for items with the fewest possible ingredients.

Foods to avoid

Fast food: French fries, cheeseburgers, hot dogs, chicken nuggets, etc.

Added sugars and sweets: Table sugar, soda, juice, pastries, cookies, candy, sweet tea, sugary cereals, etc.

Refined grains: White rice, white pasta, white bread, bagels, etc.

Packaged and convenience foods: Chips, crackers, cereal bars, frozen dinners, etc.

Processed vegan-friendly foods: Plant-based meats like Tofurkey, faux cheeses, vegan butters, etc.

Artificial sweeteners: Equal, Splenda, Sweet'N Low, etc.

Processed animal products: bacon, lunch meats, sausage, beef jerky, etc.

Fatty meat: pork, lamb, shellfish (high in saturated fat)

Foods to minimize

While healthy animal foods can be included in a WFPB diet, they should be minimized. These include:

- Beef (only lean)

- poultry

- eggs

- dairy (only low fat)

- fish

When following a WFPB diet, highly processed foods should be avoided, and animal products should be minimized.

Calorie Deficit and Intermittent Fasting

Understanding how cutting calories and intermittent fasting work can really help you lose weight in a healthy and lasting way.

Using these two methods together is a strong strategy for getting rid of extra weight.

When you eat fewer calories than your body uses to maintain weight, you create a calorie deficit. This causes your body to use its stored fat for energy, which leads to weight loss. But it's important to cut calories in a smart way. You need to make sure that even though you're eating less, you're still getting all the important nutrients your body needs to work well.

Intermittent fasting is when you switch between eating and not eating (fasting). This eating style can help change the way your body's hormones work, improve your metabolism (how your body turns food into energy), and help your body burn fat more easily. Adopting intermittent fasting and having fewer calories at the same time can greatly speed up your weight loss.

Research has found that intermittent fasting is a safe and effective way to lose weight. It works about as well as other diets do. Some studies suggest that eating only during a specific 8 to 10-hour period during the day, which fits our body's natural clock, can help with weight loss.

This method seems to be especially helpful for people who might be at risk of developing diabetes. But it's very important to find a way of eating that you can keep up over time and that fits well with how you live and what your body needs[8].

---

[8]https://www.health.harvard.edu/blog/intermittent-fasting-surprising-update-2018062914156

Portion Control: Building a Healthy and Balanced Diet

Creating a balanced diet is key to maintaining your health and managing your weight. Here's how you can structure your meals for balance and nutrition:

- **Vegetables and Fruits – ½ of Your Plate:** Fill half your plate with vegetables and fruits[9]. If your goal is to lose weight, start your meals with a low-calorie green-salad bowl. Dark, leafy greens like spinach, kale, arugula, and romaine are packed with fiber and make you feel fuller. The resultant increased feeling of satiety means you will likely eat fewer calories during your main course. Aim a variety of colors to ensure you're getting a range of nutrients. However, be mindful that potatoes don't count towards the healthy vegetable quota due to their impact on blood sugar.

- **Whole Grains – ¼ of Your Plate:** Choose whole grains like quinoa, oats, brown rice, and millet and buckwheat[10], legumes,whole wheat pasta , barley. Keep in mind if you like bread, look for a local bakery and buy only whole grains bread: rye or whole wheat.

Most breads available in supermarkets are highly processed with added sugar and hydrogenated oils.

- **Protein Power – ¼ of Your Plate:** Choose healthy proteins like fish (avoid fish that contains the highest levels of mercury including swordfish, mackerel, yellowtail, tuna, and sea

---

[9]https://www.hsph.harvard.edu/nutritionsource/what-should-you-eat/vegetables-and-fruits/
[10]https://www.hsph.harvard.edu/nutritionsource/what-should-you-eat/whole-grains/

bass), poultry, beans, non-fat yogurt or milk, and nuts[11]. These proteins are versatile, can be added to salads, and go well with vegetables on your plate. Try to limit red meat and avoid processed meats high in sodium like bacon and sausage.

- **Balanced Eating Throughout the Day:** Aim to have three balanced meals and 1 to 2 snacks per day. For snacks, the best options are raw nuts and fruits combined together.

- Benefits of eating fruits and nuts together include: - Balanced nutrition: Fruits provide natural sugars and vitamins, while nuts offer healthy fats, protein, fiber. - Satiety: The combination of fruits and nuts can help you feel full and satisfied due to the fiber and protein content. - Nutrient absorption: Some vitamins and minerals in fruits are better absorbed in the presence of healthy fats, which nuts provide.

- Risks are minimal, but it's important to be mindful of portion sizes, especially if you're watching your calorie intake, as nuts are calorie-dense. Additionally, some people may have allergies to certain nuts, so it's important to be aware of any allergies before consuming them.

Stick to no more than one handful of nuts and two cups of fruits or one bowl of mixed berries a day. The best time to eat fruit is in the morning or afternoon. Keep in mind fruits have natural sugar, so it's best to limit them to one to two cups a day.

---

[11]https://www.hsph.harvard.edu/nutritionsource/what-should-you-eat/protein/

- **Healthy Plant Oils – In Moderation:** Use healthy vegetable oils such as olive or avocado oil[12]. Both of these are nutrient-rich but calorie-dense oils, so sticking to about 1-2 tablespoons a day makes an ideal routine. Steer clear of partially hydrogenated oils, as they contain unhealthy trans fats.

- **Stay Hydrated:** Drink 2-3 L of water, coffee (try to limit coffee intake to once a day because coffee increases cortisol levels), or herbal tea[13]. Avoid sugary drinks and juices, and limit your intake of milk and dairy products to one or three servings per week (the best option is a non-fat yogurt or milk). The full-fat dairy products are high in sodium and saturated fat, which increase bad cholesterol levels (LDL).

Reduce sodium intake

Key facts

Almost everyone in different parts of the world consume too much sodium.

The global mean intake of sodium for adults is 4310 mg/day sodium (equivalent to 10.78 g/day salt)[14]. This is more than double the World Health Organization recommendation for adults of less than 2000 mg/day sodium (equivalent to < 5 g/day salt).

---

[12]https://www.hsph.harvard.edu/nutritionsource/what-should-you-eat/fats-and-cholesterol/
[13] https://www.hsph.harvard.edu/nutritionsource/healthy-drinks/
[14] https://www.nature.com/articles/d42473-023-00278-3

According to the Dietary Guidelines for Americans, healthy individuals should consume no more than 2300 mg of sodium per day. That is about one teaspoon.

The primary health effect associated with diets high in sodium is increased blood pressure, which increases the risk of cardiovascular diseases, gastric cancer, obesity, osteoporosis, Meniere's disease, and kidney disease.

An overconsumption of sodium is associated with an estimated 1.89 million deaths each year.[15]

Keep Moving: Staying active is crucial for weight control. Incorporate physical activity into your daily routine to support your diet and maintain a healthy weight[16].

Quick Tips to Stock a Healthy Kitchen

Creating a healthy kitchen is all about making smart choices with what you stock up on. Here's how to ensure your kitchen supports your health and nutrition goals:

1. Prioritize Local Produce

- **Go Local:** Whenever possible, choose locally grown fruits and vegetables. Local produce is often fresher and more nutrient-dense.

- **Variety and Volume:** Make sure to eat plenty of vegetables every day, aiming for a rainbow of colors on your plate. Different

---

[15] https://www.paho.org/en/enlace/salt-intake
[16] https://www.hsph.harvard.edu/nutritionsource/staying-active/

colors mean different nutrients, so mixing it up ensures you get a broad range of vitamins and minerals.

2. Grains for Gains

- **Whole Over Refined:** Swap out refined grains like white rice for whole grains such as barley, bulgur, oat berries, quinoa, brown rice, millet, and buckwheat. These grains provide more nutrients and fiber, which can help with digestion and overall health.

- **Explore and Experiment:** Check out the bulk bins at your local grocery store to find a variety of whole grains. You might discover something new and tasty that's also easy to prepare.

3. Protein Power

- **Diverse Sources:** Focus on incorporating a variety of healthy proteins into your diet, including fresh fish, poultry (like chicken or turkey), tofu, eggs, or egg whites(egg yolk has a high cholesterol), beans, and nuts. These proteins are essential for building and repairing tissues, among other vital functions[17].

- **Balance Your Plate:** Always pair your proteins with a generous serving of vegetables and fruits, whole grains, and healthy fats to ensure a well-rounded and nutritious meal.

____

[17]https://www.hsph.harvard.edu/nutritionsource/what-should-you-eat/protein/

4. Favorable Fats and Oils

- **Choose Healthy cooking oils:** Cold-pressed oils like avocado (for cooking) and olive oil (for salads) offer heart-healthy fats and can enhance the flavor of your dishes[18]. Raw nuts are a perfect source of healthy fats(only half a cup a day)

- **Cooking and Dressing:** Cold-pressed avocado oil is the best option when it comes to cooking. Avocado oil may benefit health in several ways. It's a good source of fatty acids that are known to support and protect the health of the heart. Avocado oil also provides antioxidant and anti-inflammatory substances, such as carotenoids and vitamin E . Avocado oil contains plant compounds that are known to support health, including polyphenols, proanthocyanidins, and carotenoids.[2] These compounds help protect against oxidative damage and regulate inflammation in the body

Extra virgin olive oil is the best for salads. It is full of antioxidants and heart-healthy fats. It is also associated with health benefits like

- Decreased inflammation

- A lower risk of heart disease

- Protection against cancer

Other than these oils, keep in mind that olive oil with lemon juice is the best salad dressing recipe.

---

[18]https://www.hsph.harvard.edu/nutritionsource/2014/06/09/how-to-choose-healthy-fats/

By focusing on these areas when stocking your kitchen, you're setting the stage for nutritious and delicious meals that can support your health and wellness goals. Remember, the journey to a healthier lifestyle starts with what you bring into your home.

Dangers of Fast and Packaged Foods

Eating a lot of fast food and pre-packaged meals might be easy and save time, but it's not great for anyone trying to lose weight. These foods usually have a lot of unhealthy fats, extra sugar, and lots of artificial stuff that isn't good for you[19].

One big problem with fast and packaged foods is that they have too many calories that don't really give your body what it needs. These "empty calories" don't have much nutrition. In fact, they can lead to weight gain instead.

Also, because these foods are made to last longer on the shelf and taste a certain way, they have a lot of artificial ingredients like preservatives and things to make them taste better. These can cause inflammation in your body, mess with your stomach, and lead to other health problems.

Another problem with eating a lot of fast food and meals from packages is they don't have enough of the good stuff your body needs, like fiber, vitamins, and minerals. These nutrients are super important because they help keep your metabolism (how your body uses energy) working well, control how hungry you feel, and elevate your energy levels. When you don't get enough of these nutrients, you might find yourself feeling hungry all the

---

[19] https://foodinsight.org/the-science-behind-mindful-eating/

time and craving snacks that aren't good for you, making it even more difficult to accomplish your health goals.

Thus, it's best to avoid fast and packaged foods as much as possible. Making your own meals at home lets you choose what you put in your food and how much you eat, which is a great way to take care of your health and help you lose weight in a good way.

Why Only Choose Non-GMO and Organic Foods?

Choosing to eat foods that are non-GMO and organic can be a smart move when you're trying to lose weight in a healthy way. But you might be wondering why these kinds of foods are recommended.

When you pick non-GMO foods, you're choosing foods that haven't had their genes changed in a lab. Some people worry that foods changed this way might cause health problems, like allergies, diseases where the body attacks itself, or even cancer. By choosing non-GMO, you can avoid these worries and also support farming that's better for our health and the planet.

Organic foods are grown without man-made chemicals like pesticides and fertilizers, which can be bad for you. These chemicals can mess up the way your body works, make it easier to gain weight, and increase your risk of getting sick with long-lasting diseases. Eating organic foods means you're eating things that are probably healthier because the soil they grow in is healthier. It also means you're helping to keep the earth's soil and plants healthy and full of life.

Adding non-GMO and organic foods to your diet means you're focusing on eating really clean and healthy foods. These kinds of foods are full of nutrients and don't contain a lot of the bad chemicals that can be found in other foods.

When it comes to meat, organic meat is often thought to be a better choice than non-organic meat. This is because animals raised for organic meat are treated better, it's kinder to the environment, and the meat might have more good nutrients. Some studies show organic meats have more omega-3 fatty acids, which are good for your heart, and more antioxidants, which can protect your body from damage. Organic meats are also less likely to have leftover antibiotics or man-made hormones, which can be a worry for our health.

The Ugly Truth About Cooking Vegetable Oils

Vegetable oils, like soybean, corn, and canola oils, are often said to be healthier than fats like butter or lard. However, the real story about these oils is not so simple and deserves a closer look.

A lot of the vegetable oils we use have gone through a lot of processing and have trans fats in them. Trans fats are really bad for your health. They can make you gain weight, increase your chances of getting heart disease, and cause inflammation in your body. Also, making these oils usually involves strong chemicals, which means they might not be as healthy as we thought.

When these oils are used for cooking at high temperatures, they can form aldehydes. These are dangerous chemicals that can raise your risk of getting cancer and other serious health problems. So, even if you're trying to make healthier choices by using vegetable oils, you might still be putting harmful substances into your body without realizing it. This could make it tough for you to stick to your weight loss plans.

To deal with this problem, it's a good idea to start using healthier fats like olive oil for salads or avocado oil for cooking on high heat. These options don't go through as much processing and can handle heat better, making them a safer choice for your meals. Also, trying cooking methods that don't need a lot of oil, like baking, steaming, or grilling, can also help you avoid the issues that come with using vegetable oils at high temperatures.

Toxins-Free Lifestyle: EWG and Mamavation.com

Living a life without toxins is very important for keeping you healthy and feeling good. Websites like the Environmental Working Group (EWG) and Mamavation.com are great places to learn how to reduce the harmful stuff you come into contact with every day.

The EWG is a group that works hard to tell people about what's really in the products we use, from the food we eat and the makeup we wear to the cleaning products we use in our homes. They have a platform called the Skin Deep database, where you can look up what's in your beauty and personal care products. This helps you understand if these things are safe and if they could be bad for your health. Knowing this lets you choose products that are better for you and don't have any toxic chemicals.

By using resources like the EWG and Mamavation.com, you can learn a lot about how to avoid toxic products. This is a big step toward being healthier and making sure the things around you aren't going to harm your health.

Mamavation.com is another helpful website that aims to create a healthy, toxin-free living space for families. It talks about the dangers of common harmful substances found in things we use every day, like food, cleaning products, and items we use for personal care. It also gives useful tips on how to avoid these toxins. Following the advice from Mamavation.com can lead to small but impactful changes in how you and your family live, making everyone healthier.

Detox Your Body

Cleaning out the toxins from your body is a key part of improving your health. Every day, toxins enter our lives, through the air, the processed food we eat, and even from the stress we develop. These toxins can seriously harm your health. Making detoxing a part of your daily life can help your body get rid of these harmful substances.

Eating foods that are natural and not processed is a great way to help your body clean itself out. Eating different kinds of fruits, veggies, whole grains, and lean meats can really help your body eliminate these toxins. This supports your body's natural way of cleaning itself and can make you feel a lot better.

Cutting down on processed foods, sugar, and alcohol is also crucial for helping your body detox. Let's look at why it's good to eat less of these things:

Alcohol: Alcohol has a lot of calories, especially when you mix it with sweet drinks, which can lead to weight gain. It can make you hungrier and less careful about what you eat, leading you to make unhealthy food choices. Drinking too much over time can not only make you gain weight but can also mess up the balance of nutrients you need.

Drinking a lot of alcohol regularly can also harm your liver, leading to diseases like fatty liver, alcoholic hepatitis, and cirrhosis. When your liver isn't working right, it's harder for your body to process nutrients and control blood sugar, which can make you gain more weight and increase your risk of diseases like diabetes.

Processed Foods: Processed foods often have a lot of extra sugar, unhealthy fats, and processed grains that make their calorie count high but don't give you much nutrition. This can lead to consuming more calories than you burn, which might make you gain weight.

A big problem with processed foods is that they don't have enough nutrients to make you feel full, and therefore, they can lead you to overeat.

Also, processed foods are made to taste really good. They have things added to them, like flavor enhancers and artificial sweeteners, that can make your brain want more. This can make you eat too much of them and can cause weight gain.

Moreover, processed foods that have a lot of refined sugars and grains can make your blood sugar levels go up quickly. This can mess with the mechanism through which your body tells you whether you're hungry or full, making you want to eat more, possibly leading to more weight gain.

Sugar: Consuming sugar raises your blood sugar levels. This makes your pancreas release insulin, which helps convert sugar into energy. But if you eat too much sugar, you'll have a lot of insulin in your body all the time. This can make your body store fat and not break it down, which can lead to weight gain and even obesity.

Too much sugar, especially a type called fructose, can also mess up your metabolism. This can make you store fat in your liver and belly and can alter the fats in your blood in harmful ways. These changes can make you gain weight and increase your chance of getting illnesses like fatty liver disease, insulin resistance, and type 2 diabetes. Sugar can also make your brain feel good, which can make you want to eat more sugary foods.

Following these guidelines can help you build a diet that supports your health and weight management goals. Remember, the key is balance and variety, ensuring your body gets the nutrients it needs to function optimally. Plus, adding detox habits to your everyday life can set you up for long-term health success. When you help your body's natural cleaning processes, you improve your overall health and optimize your well-being.

Chapter 5: Exercise: Moving Your Body

In a world where convenience and sedentary lifestyles have become the norm, the importance of exercise has never been more crucial. Far beyond simply burning calories, the act of moving your body holds the power to transform your physical health, mental well-being, and even the very way your body metabolizes energy. Whether you're seeking to lose weight, build strength, or simply feel more vibrant and energized, the transformative effects of exercise are poised to unlock a new range of possibilities.

In this chapter, we will explore the multifaceted benefits of incorporating movement into your daily life, understand the dangers of idleness, check out the various exercising options for yourself, and uncover the strategies to create a personalized exercise regimen that will have you feeling better, inside and out.

Importance of Exercise for Metabolism

Exercise is critical to boost metabolism and help you lose weight in a healthy, long-term way. Let's take a look at how exercise affects your metabolism and how it can help you reach your weight loss goals.

Your metabolism is the process your body uses to convert the food you eat into energy. When you exercise, your body burns calories to power your moving muscles. This increases your metabolism, making it more efficient at burning calories even when you're resting, and the effects can persist for several hours after the workout.

The extent of the increase in metabolic rate depends on the intensity and duration of the exercise. Aerobic exercise, particularly vigorous aerobic exercise, can elevate your heart rate to approximately 80 percent of your maximal heart rate for at least 20 minutes, leading to an increase in calorie burn for an average of 14 hours post-exercise. High-intensity interval training (HIIT) can also produce dramatic physiological benefits, including increased aerobic capacity and fat metabolism[20].

A study published in the journal Cardiovascular Research found that the metabolic effects of exercise are more profound than previously reported. The study, which controlled for various factors such as diet, stress, sleep patterns, and work environment, revealed that exercise can increase metabolism significantly[21].

Exercises that build muscle are especially helpful for boosting metabolism. Muscle tissue requires more energy to maintain than fat tissue, so the more muscle you have, the higher your metabolism will be. Strength training exercises like weightlifting can help you build and maintain muscle mass over time. After a strenuous workout, your body begins to restore glycogen and other energy-producing components within your muscles, which requires additional energy expenditure. As you create more

---

[20]https://www.livestrong.com/article/485498-does-exercise-raise-your-metabolic-rate-for-several-hours-after-the-workout/
[21]https://www.escardio.org/The-ESC/Press-Office/Press-releases/Benefits-of-exercise-on-metabolism-more-profound-than-previously-reported

active muscle tissue from lifting weights, your resting metabolic rate increases.

Cardiovascular exercises like running, cycling, or swimming can also increase your metabolism. These workouts get your heart pumping, causing your body to burn more calories during and after the exercise.

To get the highest benefits for your metabolism, it's important to combine exercise with a healthy, balanced diet. A personalized diet plan that provides the right nutrients and calorie intake, along with a customized exercise routine, can optimize your metabolism and help you achieve sustainable weight loss.

By understanding how exercise impacts your metabolism and incorporating it into your lifestyle, you can unlock the key to long-term weight management and maintain a healthy, efficient metabolic state.

Dangers of Sedentary Lifestyle

In today's fast-paced world, many people find themselves leading increasingly sedentary lifestyles, which are characterized by prolonged periods of sitting or inactivity. This lack of physical activity can have far-reaching consequences, putting your overall health and well-being at risk. It's crucial to understand the dangers of a sedentary lifestyle and take proactive steps to incorporate more movement into your daily routine.

When you don't regularly move your body, the calories you consume are not being burned off effectively. This can lead to an excess of stored fat, ultimately resulting in weight gain and, in more severe cases, obesity. Research has shown that sedentary behavior is associated with increased body weight and obesity, even when controlling for physical activity levels[22].

A study published in the journal BMJ Open found that different types of sedentary behavior, such as television viewing and computer use, are most consistently related to higher body mass index (BMI) and large waist circumference in both sexes[23]. Another study examined the association between sedentary time and obesity in a multi-ethnic population and found that sedentary behavior was associated with increased BMI and waist circumference[24].

In addition, obesity is closely associated with a host of other health issues, including heart disease, diabetes, high blood pressure, metabolic disorders, and certain types of cancer, which can have a significant impact on your quality of life.

Staying sedentary for extended periods can also lead to muscle loss and decreased bone density due to the lack of mechanical stress on the bones and muscles. This phenomenon is related to the mechanostat theory, which suggests that both exercise and physical activity can drive direct and indirect osteogenic effects on bone mass.

Physical activity and exercise are very important for maintaining bone health throughout life. The skeleton is designed to bear the weight of your body and to provide support for your muscles. Bones and muscles are meant to be used daily.

---

[22] https://pubmed.ncbi.nlm.nih.gov/29189928/
[23] https://bmjopen.bmj.com/content/3/6/e002901
[24] https://www.ncbi.nlm.nih.gov/books/NBK565813/

If you conduct a sedentary life and don't exercise, your muscles will slowly lose strength and shrink; likewise, sitting or lying most of the day without walking or exercising will cause your bones to lose mineralized tissue and strength. Weak muscles and bones will increase the risk of a fracture.

There are two types of exercise that you can perform to keep your bones and muscles healthy: weight-bearing and muscle-strengthening[25].

Another study by Lin et al. found that sedentary activity is negatively correlated with bone density and is strongly associated with an increase in body fat percentage. Without regular physical activity, your muscles begin to weaken and deteriorate, making it more challenging to perform everyday tasks and increasing your risk of injury[26].

Prolonged sitting has also been linked to an increased risk of chronic health conditions, such as cardiovascular disease and certain types of cancer. Sedentary behavior has been identified as an independent risk factor for cancer, even among those who engage in regular exercise.

A study by the American Cancer Society found that adults who spent more than 6 hours per day sitting had a 30% higher risk of developing colon cancer compared to those who sat for less than 3 hours per day[27]. Additionally, a meta-analysis of studies by the National Cancer Institute found that sedentary behavior was

---

[25]https://bonehealth.wustl.edu/patient-care/facts-about-osteoporosis/exercise-and-bone-health

[26] https://www.nature.com/articles/s41598-023-35742-z

[27]https://cancer.ca/en/cancer-information/reduce-your-risk/move-more-sit-less/how-sedentary-behaviour-increases-your-risk-of-cancer

associated with a 28-44% increase in relative risk for colon cancer[28].

Furthermore, a study by the University of Texas MD Anderson Cancer Center found that participants with the greatest total sedentary time had a 52% increased risk of dying from cancer, with the best estimate ranging from a 1% to a 127% increased risk. The study also found that participants with the longest bouts of uninterrupted sedentary behavior had a 36% higher risk of cancer mortality compared to those with shorter bouts of sedentary behavior[29].

In terms of cardiovascular disease, a review of prospective studies found that sedentary behaviors increase the risk of cardiovascular disease, independent of physical activity[30]. The World Health Organization recommends at least 150 minutes of moderate-intensity aerobic physical activity or 75 minutes of vigorous-intensity aerobic physical activity per week to maintain a healthy lifestyle[31]. However, even light physical activity can have health benefits, as suggested by a study that found replacing 30 minutes of sedentary time per day with light activity led to a 31% lower risk of dying from cancer.

Furthermore, the lack of physical activity can have a negative impact on your mental well-being, contributing to the development of conditions like depression and anxiety.

---

[28] https://www.ncbi.nlm.nih.gov/pmc/articles/PMC7931121/
[29]https://www.medicalnewstoday.com/articles/sedentary-lifestyle-linked-to-cancer-mortality
[30] https://academic.oup.com/ije/article/41/5/1338/709862
[31] https://jamanetwork.com/journals/jamaoncology/fullarticle/2767093

To combat the dangers of a sedentary lifestyle, it's essential to incorporate regular physical activity into your daily routine. This can be as simple as taking regular breaks to stand up and stretch, going for a brisk walk during your lunch break, or engaging in activities like jogging, cycling, or swimming. By making small yet impactful changes to increase your overall activity level, you can begin to mitigate the risks associated with a sedentary lifestyle and take a proactive approach to improving your health and well-being.

Remember, the key to unlocking the benefits of a more active lifestyle is to start small and build momentum. With a commitment to regular physical activity and a balanced approach to your overall health, you can reclaim your vitality and reduce the dangers of a sedentary lifestyle.

Types of Exercise: Cardio, Strength Training, Flexibility, Stretching

Achieving sustainable weight loss requires a well-rounded approach to exercise, incorporating a variety of activities to target different aspects of your physical health. By exploring the different types of exercise and understanding how they can work together, you can create a comprehensive routine that will help you reach your weight loss goals and maintain a healthy, active lifestyle.

Cardiovascular exercises, or "cardio" for short, are renowned for their ability to burn calories and improve your overall heart health. Activities like running, cycling, swimming, and dancing elevate your heart rate, allowing you to increase your endurance and stamina. These exercises improve cardiovascular function by reducing resting heart rate, blood pressure, and chances of clogged arteries. They also make your heart muscles stronger and ensure that it gets a good supply of blood. Regular cardiovascular exercise also increases high-density lipoprotein (HDL) cholesterol levels, which can help reduce stress on the heart and improve overall cardiovascular health[32].

On top of that, engaging in regular cardio can help you burn a significant number of calories, both during and after your workout, making it a powerful tool in your weight loss arsenal.

In addition to these benefits, cardiovascular exercises have been linked to a reduced risk of developing cardiovascular diseases (CVD) in individuals who are lean, obese, or have type 2 diabetes[33]. A systematic review found that exercise-based cardiac rehabilitation improved cardiovascular function in patients with CVD, reducing CVD-related mortality, decreasing the risk of myocardial infarction, and improving quality of life.

While cardio focuses on burning calories, strength training exercises are essential for building and maintaining lean muscle mass. Activities such as weightlifting, bodyweight exercises, and resistance band workouts challenge your muscles, causing them to grow stronger. The more muscle you have, the more calories your body will burn, even at rest. Regular strength training can also improve athletic performance in sports that require speed, power, and strength and may even support endurance athletes by preserving lean muscle mass[34].

---

[32] https://www.frontiersin.org/articles/10.3389/fcvm.2019.00069/full
[33] https://www.frontiersin.org/articles/10.3389/fcvm.2019.00069/full
[34]https://www.healthline.com/health/fitness/benefits-of-strength-training

A study by Wernbom et al. compared high-frequency strength training to lower-frequency strength training and found that both training methods resulted in similar improvements in lean mass and strength after 8 weeks of training. The study involved participants with strength training experience, and the high-frequency training group trained each muscle group three times per week, while the low-frequency training group trained each muscle group once per week[35].

By incorporating strength training into your routine, you can not only improve your overall strength but also help to rev up your metabolism and support your weight loss goals.

Flexibility exercises, like yoga and pilates, play a crucial role in improving your range of motion and overall mobility. These activities can help improve your posture, balance, and joint health, which can translate to better performance during other types of exercises. Additionally, improving your flexibility can help reduce the risk of injuries, allowing you to exercise more consistently and effectively.

While often overlooked, stretching exercises are an essential component of a well-rounded fitness routine. Regular stretching can help improve your overall flexibility, reduce muscle tension, and enhance your recovery between workouts. A systematic review with meta-analysis by Behm et al. found that an acute bout of stretching can provide small but significant improvements in joint range of motion (ROM) for most ROM

---

[35] https://www.ncbi.nlm.nih.gov/pmc/articles/PMC4836564/

tests, including sit and reach, hamstrings, triceps, and hip adductor tests[36].

In addition to the acute effects, regular stretching can improve mobility over time by increasing the 'stretch tolerance' of muscles. This allows for greater movement capacity and a reduced risk of injury. Stretching also helps to maintain joint health and longevity, as well as improve athletic performance by allowing for a greater range of motion during physical activities[37].

Dynamic stretching is particularly beneficial for improving mobility and preparing the body for physical activity, while static stretching is more effective for increasing flexibility. It is recommended to incorporate both types of stretching into a regular fitness routine to achieve optimal mobility and flexibility benefits.

To achieve sustainable weight loss and maintain a healthy, active lifestyle, it's crucial to incorporate a variety of exercises into your routine. By combining cardio, strength training, flexibility, and stretching, you can create a comprehensive approach that targets different aspects of your physical health. This diversity in exercise not only helps you burn calories and build muscle but also improves your overall fitness, resilience, and long-term success in your weight loss journey.

Remember, the key is to find a balance and explore the different types of exercise to discover what works best for your individual needs and preferences. By embracing the diversity of

---

[36]https://sportsmedicine-open.springeropen.com/articles/10.1186/s40798-023-00652-x
[37] https://www.polar.com/blog/stretching-vs-mobility/

exercise, you can unlock the full potential of your weight loss journey and pave the way for a healthier, more active future.

Designing a Personalized Exercise Regimen

When it comes to achieving sustainable weight loss, designing a personalized exercise regimen is crucial. Each individual is unique, with their own fitness levels, preferences, and goals. By creating a customized exercise plan that caters to your specific needs, you can maximize the effectiveness of your workouts and make lasting progress toward your weight loss objectives.

The first step in designing your personalized exercise regimen is to assess your current fitness level and any limitations you may have. If you are new to exercise or have any medical conditions, it is highly recommended to consult with a healthcare professional before starting a new workout routine. They can help you determine the most suitable types of exercises for your body and provide guidance on how to safely increase your activity level over time.

Next, it's important to consider your fitness goals and the types of exercises that you genuinely enjoy. If you prefer high-intensity workouts, activities like running, HIIT (High-Intensity Interval Training), or cycling might be an excellent fit. On the other hand, if you prefer more low-impact activities, yoga, pilates, or swimming could be better options for you. By choosing exercises that you genuinely enjoy, you are more likely to stick with your regimen in the long run, making it a sustainable part of your lifestyle.

To prevent boredom and avoid plateauing, it is crucial to incorporate a variety of exercises into your regimen. A well-rounded approach that includes a mix of cardio, strength training, and flexibility exercises can help you target different muscle groups and keep your body challenged. Additionally, setting specific, measurable goals for your workouts can help you track your progress over time and stay motivated as you continue to push yourself.

As you embark on your personalized exercise journey, remember to listen to your body and be willing to adjust your regimen as needed. Your fitness level, goals, and preferences may change over time, and it's essential to be adaptable to ensure that your exercise plan continues to support your sustainable weight loss goals.

By designing a personalized exercise regimen that takes into account your individual needs, preferences, and goals, you can create a sustainable plan for weight loss success. Remember to start where you are, stay consistent, and be open to making adjustments as you progress. With a tailored approach, you can unlock the full potential of exercise and achieve your weight loss objectives.

As you've discovered throughout this chapter, exercise is not just about shedding pounds or building muscle – it's about unlocking a world of benefits that can positively transform every aspect of your life. From boosting your metabolism and improving your cardiovascular health to elevating your mood and enhancing your overall well-being, the power of movement is truly remarkable.

Now, armed with the knowledge and strategies to design a personalized exercise plan, the choice is yours. Will you answer the call to move your body and embark on a journey toward a healthier, happier you? The path may not always be easy, but the rewards that await are truly life-changing. So, take that first step, and let the transformative magic of exercise guide you toward a future filled with vitality, strength, and a renewed zest for living.

Chapter 6: Mindset: Cultivating a Healthy Mind

This chapter invites you on a journey to explore the inner workings of your thoughts and feelings. Just as you care for your body by eating right and exercising, your mind also needs attention and care to stay healthy and strong. This chapter is your guide to understanding how your thoughts shape your reality and how, by adopting a positive and mindful approach, you can transform challenges into opportunities for growth.

Impact of a Healthy Mindset on Goal Achievement

When it comes to reaching your weight loss goals, having a healthy mindset is absolutely crucial. Your mindset - the way you think and feel about yourself and your goals - can either push you forward toward success or hold you back from reaching your full potential. In the journey toward sustainable, long-term weight loss, maintaining a positive and healthy mindset is the key to making real progress.

If you approach your weight loss goals with a healthy, optimistic mindset, you are much more likely to stay motivated and focused on your objectives, even when the going gets tough. It's true that losing weight and getting healthier is not always easy. There will be obstacles and setbacks along the way. But when you have a positive, can-do attitude, you'll be better equipped to overcome those challenges.

By truly believing in yourself and your ability to make positive changes, you are setting yourself up for success from the very beginning. You'll be less likely to get discouraged or give up when the process gets difficult. Instead, you'll be able to push through with determination and confidence, knowing that you have what it takes to reach your goals.

A healthy mindset also plays a big role in shaping the everyday choices you make when it comes to your diet and lifestyle. When you have a positive outlook on your weight loss journey, you are more likely to make healthier decisions about the foods you eat and the amount of physical activity you get.

For example, if you view your weight loss as a chore or a punishment, you might be tempted to turn to unhealthy "comfort" foods or skip your workouts whenever you're feeling stressed or discouraged. But if you see your journey as an opportunity to take great care of your body and improve your overall health and well-being, you'll be more motivated to choose nutritious, whole foods and stick to a regular exercise routine.

Positive psychology, which focuses on the study of what makes life worth living, has been linked to healthy nutrition and positive health outcomes. Studies have found that happier people tend to be more flexible and resilient, making it easier for them to modify unhealthy habits and cope with stress[38]. A positive mindset can also help individuals focus on the variety of healthy foods available rather than a rigid diet based on exclusion.

---

[38] https://www.tutorhunt.com/resource/23904/

Food optimism, a concept that combines a positive mindset with a flexible approach to healthy eating, can lead to more enjoyable and lasting changes in dietary habits. This approach emphasizes the importance of not only healthy behaviors but also a positive mindset in promoting long-term health[39].

Research has also shown that a healthy diet can improve brain function through processes such as neurogenesis and synaptic plasticity[40]. A positive mindset can contribute to the adoption of a healthy diet, which in turn can lead to better brain function and overall well-being.

This can make all the difference in helping you achieve long-term, sustainable weight loss results. When your mindset is focused on developing healthy habits that you can maintain for life rather than quick fixes, you'll be much more likely to see real, lasting change.

Speaking of sustainable weight loss, a healthy mindset is key to avoiding the dreaded "yo-yo" effect, where you lose weight only to gain it all back (and then some) shortly after. This happens all too often when people approach weight loss in an unsustainable way, either by drastically restricting their calories or following overly restricted diets.

But when you have a healthy, balanced mindset, you'll be able to develop an approach to weight loss that you can stick to for the long haul. Instead of thinking of it as a temporary "diet, " you'll see it as a permanent lifestyle change, one that involves

---

[39]https://www.thepublicopinion.com/story/lifestyle/2018/04/02/food-optimism-how-a-positive-mindset-improves-your-relationship-with-food/44549375/
[40]https://kids.frontiersin.org/articles/10.3389/frym.2021.578214

making gradual, sustainable adjustments to your eating and exercise habits.

This might mean focusing on adding more nutritious, whole foods to your diet rather than just cutting out entire food groups. Or it could mean finding physical activities that you genuinely enjoy, rather than forcing yourself to do workouts that feel like a chore. With the right mindset, you'll be able to build healthy habits that become second nature rather than feeling like a constant struggle.

The impact of a healthy mindset on your ability to achieve your weight loss goals cannot be overstated. By cultivating a positive, can-do attitude, you'll set yourself up for long-term success not just in weight loss but in all areas of your health and well-being.

When you believe in yourself and your ability to make meaningful changes, you'll be empowered to take action and stick with it, even when the road gets tough. You'll be less likely to get discouraged by setbacks and more likely to celebrate your progress and successes along the way.

Self-talk, Belief System, Resilience

This section comprises a detailed discussion about the critical role that our mindset and mental resilience play in achieving sustainable weight loss. As we'll explore, our inner dialogue, belief system, and ability to bounce back from challenges are all essential ingredients for long-term success on our health and wellness journey.

One of the key factors that can make or break our weight loss efforts is the way we talk to ourselves and the beliefs we have about our own capabilities. Negative self-talk and limiting beliefs can be real roadblocks, undermining our motivation and causing us to give up when the going gets tough.

Negative self-talk is the inner voice that criticizes and undermines our abilities, often leading to feelings of helplessness, stress, and decreased motivation[41]. This type of self-talk can create a vicious cycle, where the negative thoughts reinforce the belief that we are incapable or unworthy, which in turn affects our interpretation of the world around us and our ability to achieve our goals.

Limiting beliefs, on the other hand, are deeply ingrained internal beliefs that we take as absolute truths about our capabilities, the world, and our interactions with others. These beliefs often stem from childhood experiences, family beliefs, and life experiences and can be rooted in emotions that are not based on actual evidence. Limiting beliefs can prevent us from straying from our comfort zone, as they act as a defense from hurt and disappointment, but at the cost of preventing us from achieving our goals[42].

For example, if we constantly tell ourselves things like "I'll never be able to stick to a healthy eating plan" or "I don't have the willpower to lose weight, " those messages will become self-

---

[41]https://www.verywellmind.com/negative-self-talk-and-how-it-affects-us-4161304
[42]https://www.embracesexualwellness.com/esw-blog/2023/6/8/how-to-manage-limiting-beliefs-and-negative-self-talk

fulfilling assumptions. Our mindset will become a barrier to the very changes we're trying to make.

The consequences of negative self-talk and limiting beliefs can be significant, including a higher risk of mental health problems, increased stress, reduced success, and a host of other damaging effects. These negative thoughts and beliefs can also lead to a lowered ability to see opportunities and a decreased tendency to capitalize on them, further perpetuating the cycle of negativity.

To overcome these roadblocks, it is essential to recognize and challenge negative self-talk and limiting beliefs. This can be done by being intentional about noticing which negative thoughts and beliefs come up habitually, making a list of these recurring thoughts, and identifying their origins. Cognitive-behavioral therapy (CBT) can be an effective tool in addressing negative self-talk and limiting beliefs, as it involves restructuring how we think and perceive the world around us[43].

On the flip side, cultivating a positive and empowering belief system can be a game-changer. When we talk to ourselves with compassion and encouragement and truly believe in our ability to achieve our goals, we're setting ourselves up for success. We'll be more likely to persevere through challenges, bounce back from slip-ups, and stay motivated and focused in the long term.

A crucial part of developing a healthy, positive mindset is practicing self-compassion. Instead of beating ourselves up over

---

[43]https://beautifulsoulcounseling.com/overcoming-negative-self-talk-and-limiting-beliefs/

mistakes or setbacks, we can choose to treat ourselves with kindness and understanding.

It's human nature to stumble and fall short sometimes, especially when we're trying to make big changes in our lives. But far too often, we are our own harshest critics. We berate ourselves for not being "perfect" or for not sticking to our plans 100% of the time.

However, research shows that self-compassion, the ability to be gentle, understanding, and forgiving with ourselves, is a much more effective and sustainable approach. When we can look at our slip-ups with self-love and recognize that we're all a work in progress, we're more likely to get right back on track, learn from our mistakes, and keep moving forward.

In addition to a positive belief system and self-compassion, resilience is another essential trait for achieving long-term weight loss success. Life is full of ups and downs, and when we're on a health and wellness journey, we're bound to face obstacles and setbacks along the way.

Whether it's dealing with cravings, navigating social situations that challenge our healthy habits, or bouncing back from a stalled weight loss, resilience is what will keep us going. It's the ability to face the storms head-on, learn from our challenges, and emerge stronger on the other side.

Building resilience might involve developing effective coping strategies, such as stress management techniques or seeking support from loved ones. It could also mean practicing mindfulness, which can help us stay grounded and focused even when things get tough.

Ultimately, resilience is about having the mental and emotional resources to bounce back, adapt, and keep moving forward, no matter what life throws our way. And when we cultivate that kind of resilience, it becomes a powerful asset in our weight loss journey and beyond.

By focusing on our self-talk, belief system, and resilience, we can create a solid foundation for sustainable weight loss and lasting lifestyle changes. When we have the right mindset in place, we're empowered to overcome any obstacles that come our way and stay committed to our health and wellness goals.

It's important to remember that weight loss is not just about the number on the scale - it's about creating a balanced, healthy lifestyle that we can maintain for the long haul.

By addressing these key aspects of your mindset, you'll be laying the foundation for sustainable, lasting change. You'll be able to overcome challenges, stay motivated, and develop healthy habits that become second nature. Ultimately, you'll be empowered to achieve your weight loss goals and maintain a healthy, balanced lifestyle for years to come.

Overcoming Limiting Beliefs and Developing a Positive Mindset

Overcoming limiting beliefs and developing a positive mindset are crucial components of achieving sustainable weight loss. Many people struggle with negative self-talk and limiting beliefs that prevent them from reaching their health and fitness goals. In order to make lasting changes, it is essential to address these mental barriers and cultivate a more empowering, positive mindset.

One of the most common limiting beliefs when it comes to weight loss is the idea that it's simply impossible or too difficult to achieve. This negative, defeatist mindset can disrupt your efforts before you even begin. You might tell yourself things like, "I'll never be able to lose weight, " or "Healthy eating is just too hard for me."

However, by challenging these limiting beliefs and replacing them with more positive, empowering thoughts, you can start to shift your mindset toward possibility and potential. Instead of focusing on all the reasons you can't succeed, try reframing your self-talk to emphasize what's possible. Remind yourself of past successes, celebrate small wins, and affirm your ability to make meaningful, lasting changes.

Developing a positive, healthy mindset also involves practicing self-compassion and self-care. It's so easy to be overly harsh and critical of ourselves, especially when we experience setbacks or slip-ups on our weight loss journeys. But constantly beating ourselves up is counterproductive and can actually undermine our progress.

Instead, we need to learn to treat ourselves with the same kindness and understanding that we would show a dear friend. When we make a "mistake" or struggle to stick to our healthy habits, we can acknowledge those feelings with compassion, without judgment. By staying present and mindful, we can learn to appreciate our bodies and all that they do for us rather than focusing solely on the areas we want to change.

This shift in mindset can make a world of difference in our ability to bounce back from challenges, stay motivated, and keep moving forward on our weight loss journey. Self-compassion helps us avoid the cycle of self-criticism and self-denial and, instead, empowers us to embrace the process of change with kindness and patience.

Self-compassion is defined as the ability to show kindness and understanding to oneself in times of suffering or failure rather than engaging in self-criticism or self-judgment. It is a practice that involves treating oneself with the same compassion and understanding that one would offer to a friend in times of difficulty or suffering[44].

Research has shown that practicing self-compassion can significantly reduce self-criticism. In a review of 19 self-compassion studies, the results showed that practicing self-compassion significantly reduces self-criticism[45].

Self-compassion has also been found to significantly reduce feelings of loneliness, as it is one of the key predictors of loneliness. Individuals high in self-compassion are less sensitive to rejection, which can help mitigate the negative effects of social rejection.

Self-compassion is different from self-esteem, which can be contingent on external factors such as physical appearance or social comparisons. Self-compassion, on the other hand, focuses

---

[44]https://cptsdfoundation.org/2024/02/01/the-antidote-for-self-criticism/
[45]https://centerformsc.org/self-compassion-and-quality-of-life-research/

on self-kindness and acceptance over self-judgment, offering a gentle way to guide oneself back to one's true self[46].

Incorporating self-compassion practices into one's life can lead to improved overall wellness, including mental, physical, social, and emotional health. It can also lead to a path of positive self-discovery, healing, and increased self-confidence[47].

Another key aspect of cultivating a positive mindset for sustainable weight loss is setting realistic, achievable goals and celebrating the progress you make along the way. It's easy to get caught up in focusing on the end result - the "perfect" weight or body image we have in mind. But when we do that, we can lose sight of the smaller, incremental changes that are just as important.

By setting realistic, incremental goals and acknowledging even the smallest victories, we can stay motivated and inspired to keep going. Maybe it's celebrating the fact that you've added an extra 10 minutes of activity to your daily routine or that you've made it through a challenging social event without derailing your healthy eating habits. Whatever the milestone, taking the time to recognize your progress can help reinforce your positive mindset and keep you moving forward.

With personalized diet plans and a focus on mindset transformation, achieving and maintaining a healthy weight becomes not only possible but enjoyable. You'll be equipped with the tools and strategies to overcome any obstacles, stay

---

[46] https://raywilliams.ca/self-criticism-self-compassion-works-best/
[47] https://www.linkedin.com/pulse/how-less-self-critical-more-self-compassionate-tina-marie?trk=articles_directory

motivated, and develop healthy habits that become second nature.

So, if you're ready to embark on a weight loss journey that will truly change your life, start by taking a close look at your mindset. What beliefs are holding you back? How can you cultivate greater self-compassion and resilience? By addressing these key aspects of your mindset, you'll be laying the foundation for sustainable, lasting change.

The road to weight loss may not always be easy, but by transforming your mindset, you'll have the power to overcome any challenge and achieve your health and wellness goals. Your healthier, happier future self is waiting - all you have to do is believe in the possibilities.

Chapter 7: Stress Management: Finding Balance

In our fast-paced world, stress has become a constant companion for many of us, impacting our lives in several ways. Yet, its effects on our health, particularly in relation to weight and well-being, are often underestimated. This chapter covers the complicated relationship between stress, health, and weight management, providing you with valuable insights and practical strategies to manage stress effectively.

By understanding and addressing the root causes of stress, we can significantly enhance our overall health, start a successful weight loss journey, and achieve a balanced, fulfilling life.

Understanding Stress and its Effects on Hormones and Mental Health

Stress is something that happens to everyone, and it's a normal part of life. However, what many people don't realize is just how deeply stress can affect us - it can mess with our hormones, change how we feel mentally, and even make losing weight more difficult.

Let's break it down a bit. When we're stressed, our bodies respond by releasing a hormone called cortisol, which is often called the "stress hormone." Cortisol has many important roles in our bodies. It helps manage how we use carbohydrates, fats, and proteins. It keeps our blood sugar levels stable and controls inflammation. All of these are good things when cortisol levels are balanced.

But when stress becomes constant, our cortisol levels can stay high for too long. This imbalance isn't good for our health and can lead to several problems. For one, it can make us hungry, especially for foods that aren't good for us, like those high in sugar and fat. It's like our bodies are preparing for a fight or flight situation by craving quick energy sources, even though we're not actually going to run away from or fight anything.

These high levels of cortisol can also slow down our metabolism, which is how fast our bodies turn food into energy. When our metabolism slows down, we burn calories more slowly. Plus, cortisol can cause our bodies to store more fat, especially around the stomach area. This type of fat is not just about how we look; it's linked to more health risks than fat stored in other parts of the body.

Stress can also have a significant impact on other hormones, particularly adrenaline and thyroid hormones, which can affect our mental feelings and make it difficult to lose weight. When we experience stress, our bodies release hormones like adrenaline (epinephrine) to help us cope with the stressful situation. Chronic stress can lead to prolonged elevation of these hormones, which can interfere with the complex feedback system that regulates the production of the thyroid hormone.[48]

In response to stress, adrenaline is also quickly released from the adrenal glands. When this happens, your palms may get sweaty, and your heart starts racing as more blood gets to the brain and muscles, thereby increasing blood pressure.

---

[48] https://www.thyforlife.com/stress-on-thyroid-function/

Essentially, you become more alert and gain more energy to deal with the stressor (or perceived threat) in the moment.[49] Chronic stress can lead to prolonged elevation of these stress hormones, impacting various bodily functions and organs, including the thyroid.

Stress can also affect the thyroid indirectly by contributing to unhealthy coping mechanisms like poor dietary choices, inadequate sleep, and physical inactivity. These factors, in turn, can affect the thyroid and worsen existing issues or contribute to the development of thyroid disorders. Moreover, stress-related hormonal changes can influence the delicate balance of sex hormones, which may indirectly affect thyroid function.[50]

So, even if you're eating healthy foods and exercising, high stress and cortisol levels can make it much harder to lose weight. It's like trying to pedal a bike uphill with the brakes on. This doesn't mean all hope is lost. Recognizing the role stress plays in our weight and overall health is the first step toward managing it.

Being stressed all the time messes with your body in other ways, too. It can make you feel really down or anxious, change your mood a lot, and make it harder for you to stick to your weight loss plan. It's really important to deal with stress so you can lose weight in a healthy way and feel better overall.

When you're stressed for a long time, it can change how your body works in ways that make you gain weight. For example, you

---

[49] https://www.thyforlife.com/stress-on-thyroid-function/
[50] https://www.india.com/health/how-stress-can-impact-the-functioning-of-thyroid-gland-expert-reveals-6598554/

might start to have problems with insulin, which is what helps control your sugar levels. This problem, called insulin resistance, means your body can't use insulin the right way. Because of this, you might start storing more fat, especially around your belly. This kind of fat storage is not just about how you look; it's linked to more serious health problems like type 2 diabetes and heart disease.

The changes that stress causes in how your body handles insulin can also make your sugar levels go up and down in ways that aren't good for you. This can make you gain more weight and have a higher chance of getting diabetes and heart disease. It's like a cycle where stress makes these health problems more likely, and then these problems can make you even more stressed.

Knowing how stress, your body's hormones, and how you feel inside are all linked together helps you find ways to handle stress better. You can try calming activities like meditation and yoga, make sure you move and exercise often, and eat healthy foods. Adding ways to deal with stress into your plan for losing weight helps you succeed over the long haul.

This isn't just about losing weight; it's about feeling good overall and being healthy. By focusing on reducing stress as part of your weight loss journey, you're more likely to keep the weight off and feel better in both your body and mind.

Strategies for Stress Reduction: Breathing Exercises, Yoga, Meditation

When you're trying to lose weight, it's really important to manage stress. Stress doesn't just make us feel upset or anxious; it can also make it harder for us to lose weight. In this section, we're going to look at different ways to help reduce stress, like breathing exercises, yoga, and meditation.

Breathing exercises are an easy but powerful way to help you feel more relaxed. When you concentrate on taking slow, deep breaths, your body starts to calm down. This not only makes you feel better but can also help with your weight loss goals.

Some breathing exercises, like the SKY Breath Meditation, have been found to be effective in reducing stress both in the short and long term. Studies have shown that these exercises engage the parasympathetic nervous system, which is responsible for the body's "rest and digest" activities, helping individuals calm down and think rationally in the face of stress[51]. Hence, adding breathing exercises to your daily life can make a big difference in handling stress.

Yoga is also great for reducing stress. The slow movements focus on breathing, and staying present can help you let go of tension and quiet your thoughts. Doing yoga regularly can boost how good you feel overall and help you get along better with your body and mind.

Hatha yoga, in particular, has been found to significantly reduce stress, anxiety, and depression in women. A study

---

[51]https://hbr.org/2020/09/research-why-breathing-is-so-effective-at-reducing-stress

showed that 12 sessions of regular hatha yoga practice led to significant reductions in stress, anxiety, and depression[52]. Other studies have also confirmed the positive effects of yoga on anxiety and depression.

Meditation is all about giving your mind a focus and getting rid of distractions. If you make some time every day to sit quietly and meditate, you can help yourself feel more at peace and lower your stress. There's a lot of proof that meditation is good for you—it can make you less anxious, boost your mood, and make you feel better overall.

Meditation can take many forms and be combined with various spiritual practices to achieve the most benefits, including lowering stress, improving immune function, and slowing mental aging. All you need to do is sit in a relaxed position and clear your mind or focus on one thought while clearing it of all others. The practice affects the body in the opposite way that stress does, triggering the body's relaxation response and restoring the body to a calm state[53].

If you make breathing exercises, yoga, and meditation part of your everyday life, you'll find it easier to deal with stress, which can also help you with your goals to lose weight. Taking good care of how you feel inside is a big step toward being successful in losing weight and staying healthy.

---

[52] https://www.ncbi.nlm.nih.gov/pmc/articles/PMC5843960/
[53] https://www.verywellmind.com/meditation-4157199

Chapter 8: Sleep Hygiene: Prioritizing Rest

Chapter 8 of "Healthy You" talks about how important good sleep is for getting and maintaining a healthy weight. Making sure you get enough rest is key for feeling good overall and for helping you lose weight. This is what sleep hygiene is all about.

"Sleep hygiene" refers to the habits you have that help you sleep well. Getting the right amount of sleep is crucial not just for staying energized and in a good mood but also for managing your weight. Studies have found that not getting enough sleep can mess with your hormones, making you hungrier and more likely to crave junk food.

If you want to focus on getting better sleep, try these tips:

1. Keep a Regular Sleep Schedule: Try to go to bed and wake up at the same time every day, even on the weekends. This helps your body get into a routine.

2. Develop a Relaxing Bedtime Routine: Doing calming activities before bed can help your body know it's time to sleep. You might read, take a warm bath, or do some gentle breathing exercises.

3. Make Your Bedroom Perfect for Sleeping: Keep your room cool, dark, and quiet. Investing in a comfy mattress and bedding can also make a big difference in how well you sleep.

4. Cut Down on Screen Time Before Bed: The blue light from phones, tablets, and computers can make it harder for you to fall asleep. Try to turn off these devices a bit before it's time to sleep.

5. Watch What You Eat and Drink Before Bed: Try to avoid caffeine, big meals, and alcohol before you go to sleep. These can all mess with your ability to get a good night's rest.

Focusing on getting enough rest and better sleep can really help with losing weight and keeping yourself healthy. It's important to remember that losing weight in a healthy way means making small changes that you can keep up with over time.

Importance of a Stable Sleep Regimen

On the path to lasting weight loss, something people often don't think much about is how important regular sleep is. Sleep really matters for our health and how we feel every day, and it also plays a big part in losing weight and maintaining a good weight in the long run.

Studies have found that not getting enough sleep can mess up the hormones that control hunger. This means you might start wanting more junk food and end up eating too much. Not sleeping enough can also slow down your metabolism, which is how your body turns food into energy. When your metabolism isn't working well, it's harder for your body to burn off calories. This can lead to gaining weight over time, which makes it tougher to stick to your weight loss plans.

Having a regular sleep schedule can help a lot with your efforts to lose weight and make you healthier overall. Try to sleep for 7-9 hours each night, as health experts suggest. Build a bedtime routine that calms you down and helps you get ready for sleep, like reading, taking a nice bath, or doing some meditation.

Staying away from things like caffeine and not using your phone or computer right before you go to bed can really help you sleep better. Also, it's good to try and sleep and wake up at the same time every day, even on weekends. This helps your body get into a rhythm and can make your sleep better overall.

Making sure you have a regular sleeping pattern can really change how well you do with losing weight. By making sure you get enough sleep and treating it as an essential part of your day, you help your body work better. This can help you a lot with reaching your weight loss goals and keeping the weight off for good.

Some of the benefits of sleep hygiene include:

1. Better sleep quality leads to better weight management: Quality sleep is essential for regulating hormones responsible for appetite control, such as ghrelin and leptin. Leptin signals satiety, while ghrelin stimulates appetite. Poor sleep can disrupt the balance of these hormones, leading to increased appetite and weight gain[54].

2. Improved mood and reduced stress: Quality sleep can help improve mood and reduce stress, which can positively impact overall mental health. Stress and negative emotions can lead to unhealthy eating habits and weight gain.

3. Enhanced immune system function: Adequate sleep helps strengthen the immune system, making it more effective in

---

[54]https://seermedical.com/blog/sleep-hygiene-what-is-it-and-why-does-it-matter/

fighting off infections and diseases. A strong immune system can help prevent illnesses that may lead to weight loss or gain.

4. Reduced risk of serious illnesses and health issues: Good sleep hygiene can help reduce the risk of developing chronic health conditions, such as obesity, diabetes, and cardiovascular diseases, which are all associated with weight issues.

5. Increased productivity and better relationships: Quality sleep can improve cognitive function, memory, and overall brain health, leading to increased productivity and better relationships, which can positively impact weight management[55].

Effects of Poor Sleep on Weight and Health

In this section, we explore how getting good sleep is really important for controlling your weight. A lot of people don't realize how not sleeping enough can affect their health and efforts to lose weight.

Studies have found that not sleeping well can mess up how your body uses energy and controls hormones, which can make you gain weight and cause other health problems. When we don't sleep enough, our bodies make more of the hormone ghrelin, which makes us feel hungry, and less of the hormone leptin, which helps us feel full. This can make us want to eat more, especially junk food, and this can lead to weight gain.

Not getting enough sleep can also make you feel more stressed, which isn't good for weight loss. When we're tired, we

---

[55]https://www.baptisthealth.com/blog/health-and-wellness/why-is-sleep-hygiene-important

often want to eat things like sweets or fatty foods because they seem like they'll give us a quick pick-me-up. But eating like this can lead to gaining weight you didn't want over time.

Plus, when you don't sleep well, you don't have much energy. This makes it difficult to motivate yourself to work out or choose healthy foods, which can start a cycle of excessive weight gain and sluggishness.

The effects of poor sleep can be summarized in the following points:

1. Hormonal imbalances: Sleep deprivation can lead to imbalances in hormones that regulate appetite, such as ghrelin and leptin. Ghrelin stimulates appetite, while leptin signals satiety. Poor sleep can disrupt the balance of these hormones, leading to increased appetite and weight gain[56].

2. Increased caloric intake: Poor sleep quality has been associated with poor food choices and increased caloric intake. Sleep-deprived individuals may be more likely to consume high-calorie, nutrient-poor foods, which can contribute to weight gain.

3. Reduced physical activity: Sleep deprivation can lead to decreased physical activity, as individuals may feel too tired or lack the motivation to exercise[57]. This can result in a lower metabolic rate and weight gain.

4. Impaired glucose tolerance and insulin sensitivity: Poor sleep quality has been linked to decreased glucose tolerance and

---

[56] https://www.ncbi.nlm.nih.gov/pmc/articles/PMC9783730/
[57] https://www.healthline.com/health-news/why-poor-sleep-can-lead-to-weight-gain

insulin sensitivity, which can contribute to weight gain and the development of obesity[58].

5. Increased stress: Poor sleep can increase stress levels, which can lead to unhealthy eating habits and weight gain. Stress can also disrupt the balance of hormones that regulate appetite, further contributing to weight gain.

To fight off the negative impact of not sleeping enough on your weight and health, it's super important to make sure you get good sleep every night. Getting into a regular sleep schedule, having a bedtime routine that helps you relax, and making your sleeping environment comfortable are all ways to sleep better.

Understanding how much sleep matters for maintaining our health and staying in shape helps us make better choices about our rest. This way, we're more likely to do well with our weight loss plans in the long run.

Factors Affecting Sleep Quality

Getting good sleep is really important for staying healthy and losing weight in a way that lasts. There are many things that can change how well you sleep, and these changes can make your journey to lose weight harder. Knowing what these things are can help you change your habits to sleep better and reach your weight loss goals.

Stress is one big thing that can mess with how well you sleep. If you're very stressed, you might find it hard to fall asleep, stay asleep, or feel really rested when you wake up. Finding good

---

[58] https://www.ncbi.nlm.nih.gov/pmc/articles/PMC3632337/

ways to deal with stress, like meditating, working out, or doing deep breathing exercises, can improve your sleep.

What you eat and drink can also change how you sleep. Drinking caffeine or alcohol or eating a lot right before bed can make it hard for you to sleep well. It's a good idea to not have these things late in the day and to eat lighter, healthier meals in the evening to help you sleep better.

In conclusion, getting a good night's sleep is really important for staying healthy and losing weight in a way that lasts. There are many things that can change how well you sleep, and these changes can make a difference to your overall health. Knowing what these things are can help you change your habits to sleep better and reach your weight loss goals.

Chapter 9: Body Image and Self-Care: Honoring Your Body

As we work toward achieving sustainable weight loss, it's really important to look beyond just the number on the scale and to start truly taking care of our bodies. How we see ourselves and how we treat ourselves can greatly affect our success in losing and maintaining weight.

Every one of us has a unique body that deserves care and respect. Rather than chasing a perfect look that might not be right for us, we should focus on feeding our bodies healthy foods, staying active, and doing things that make us feel good overall.

The first step to really respecting your body is to develop a positive view of yourself. Accept your body as it is, with all its quirks, and appreciate all the amazing things it does for you every day. It's important to love and feel compassion for yourself and to know that you are lovable and deserving of respect, no matter your body's size or shape.

Self-care is also key to taking good care of your body. This means getting plenty of sleep, finding effective ways to manage stress, drinking enough water, and doing things that make you happy and relaxed. Looking after your mental and emotional health is just as important as physical health. By making time for self-care, you not only improve your well-being but also support your journey toward a healthier weight.

By focusing on how you see yourself and taking good care of your body, you'll not only start feeling better about yourself, but you'll also be on the right path to long-term success in your weight loss efforts. Remember, losing weight for good isn't just about dropping pounds; it's about building a healthy and balanced way of living that respects your body and boosts your overall health.

In this chapter, we'll go into more detail about practical ways to feel positive about your body and how to look after yourself every day. We'll give you personalized advice and tools that will support you as you work toward sustainable weight loss and better health.

Relationship Between Self-Esteem and Body Image

The way we feel about our bodies and our overall self-esteem are deeply connected, and this can be confusing and tough to handle. Many people find their self-esteem takes a hit when they see their bodies negatively, which can start a cycle of criticizing themselves and feeling bad about how they look. In my book, "Healthy You, " I talk about how important it is to understand this connection and how it affects your efforts to lose weight.

It's very important to realize that self-esteem and your perception of your body go hand in hand. If someone doesn't feel good about themselves, they might not feel good about their body either. This can lead them to eat poorly and lack the motivation to make healthy changes. But people who feel good about themselves usually feel better about their bodies and are more likely to take care of themselves.

According to a study, there are gender differences in body image and self-esteem. Women tend to have lower self-esteem and more negative body image than men[59]. Personality types also play a role in both body image and self-esteem. For instance, people with high levels of self-esteem are more likely to have a positive body image, while those with low self-esteem are more likely to have a negative body image.

Social physique anxiety (SPA) is a psychological construct that encompasses the fear of negative evaluation by others based on one's body shape and appearance. SPA has been linked to both body image and self-esteem, as individuals with higher levels of SPA tend to have more negative body images and lower self-esteem.

Social media, in particular, can have a significant impact on self-esteem and body image. The perpetuation of idealized images and beauty standards can lead to feelings of inadequacy and dissatisfaction with one's own appearance, contributing to negative body image and low self-esteem. Negative comments and cyberbullying on social media can also harm self-esteem and body image, as individuals may internalize these criticisms and feel inadequate or insecure about their appearance[60].

Improving your self-esteem and how you see your body is a big part of losing weight in a way that lasts. Working on feeling more confident and valuing yourself can help you have a better relationship with your body and make lasting, healthy changes in your life. This can mean taking care of yourself, setting goals that

---

[59]https://esource.dbs.ie/server/api/core/bitstreams/fbb3fbd3-ad8a-4f9a-a804-476a0e321eb6/content
[60]https://www.linkedin.com/pulse/impact-social-media-self-esteem-body-image-samhita-bhattacharya

are realistic, and choosing to be around positive people and influences.

In my book, I offer diet plans that are tailored to fit each person's specific needs and likes. I focus on the emotional parts of losing weight, like how we feel about ourselves and how we see our bodies. My aim is to help people succeed over the long term on their path to lasting weight loss.

The connection between how we feel about ourselves and how we see our bodies is really important in whether we succeed in losing weight. By understanding and improving these areas and by making positive changes to boost self-esteem, people can build a strong base. This helps them not only lose weight for good but also improve their overall health and happiness.

Practicing Self-Love and Self-Care

In the process of losing weight in a way that lasts, it's very important to practice self-love and self-care, but these aspects often don't get enough attention. Many people focus just on the physical sides of weight loss, like eating right and exercising, and forget about the mental and emotional sides. However, loving yourself and taking good care of yourself is the key to keeping weight off for good.

Self-love means accepting and valuing yourself as you are, no matter your size or shape. It's about being kind to yourself instead of always feeling bad because you don't fit certain hard-to-reach standards. When you love yourself, you can stop negative thoughts about yourself and start seeing your body in a positive light. This positive body image is really important for losing weight and keeping it off.

Self-care is about looking after your whole well-being—your body, mind, and emotions. This includes sleeping enough, managing stress, doing things that make you happy, and setting limits with others. When you make self-care a priority, you're in a better position to make healthy choices and keep up with your weight loss plan.

Self-care practices, including self-reflection and emotional expression, contribute to better emotional regulation. Self-love, on the other hand, can help individuals understand their worth and value as a person, reducing the need for reminders or reassurance from others[61]. Moreover, self-care can increase energy levels and improve mood, which are essential for staying motivated and optimistic[62].

Adding self-love and self-care to your weight loss journey can keep you motivated, help you face challenges, and avoid getting too stressed or tired. Remember, losing weight for good isn't just about eating differently or exercising more; it's about changing how you think about and treat yourself. By embracing self-love and self-care, you lay a strong foundation for long-term success and can reach your weight loss goals in a way that's good for you.

---

[61]https://www.psychologicalhealthcare.com.au/blog/learn-to-love-yourself/
[62]https://www.linkedin.com/advice/3/how-can-you-use-self-care-stay-motivated-when-working-xtnie

Dangers of Self-Hatred

The section "Dangers of Self-Hatred" looks closely at how feeling bad about oneself can badly affect someone trying to lose weight. Self-hatred can be a big obstacle, not just for losing weight but also for maintaining overall health. Often, when people eat too much or don't look after their physical health, it's because they have deep-seated feelings of not liking themselves.

Research shows that low self-esteem, which can be a result of negative feelings about oneself, is associated with poorer weight loss outcomes[63]. One explanation is that negative body image, which is often linked to low self-esteem, can lead to unhealthy eating behaviors and poor dietary choices, hindering weight loss efforts. Individuals with low self-esteem may turn to emotional eating, consuming high-calorie foods to cope with negative emotions, which can hinder weight loss goals[64].

One of the biggest problems with self-hatred is the cycle of shame and guilt it creates. If you keep criticizing yourself for not meeting your goals or for making mistakes, it can start a harmful cycle where you sabotage your own efforts. This constant negative talk can make it really hard to keep up with your weight loss plans and can stop you from making positive, long-term changes in how you live.

Moreover, hating yourself can lead to unhealthy ways of eating, like binge eating or going on extreme diets. These habits can hurt your body and mind, leading to a lack of important

---

[63]https://karger.com/ofa/article/16/3/293/835954/Weight-Loss-History-and-Its-Association-with-Self
[64] https://ojs.lib.uwo.ca/index.php/hucjilm/article/download/7868/6484

nutrients, messed-up hormones, and a higher chance of developing eating disorders.

To escape the harmful effects of self-hatred, it's really important to learn to be kind to yourself and love yourself. Building a good relationship with yourself can help you feel worthy and powerful, which can help a lot on your weight loss journey. This means you need to fight against negative thoughts, take good care of yourself, and get support from friends, family, or maybe a therapist.

By dealing with the problems caused by self-hatred and encouraging kindness to oneself, you can lay a strong foundation for successfully losing weight and keeping it off. It's very important to understand that true change happens when you accept and love yourself, not when you dislike yourself.

Embracing Your Body Image

In a world where there are often very tough and unrealistic expectations about how we should look, it can be hard to feel good about your own body. However, learning to accept and appreciate your body is a key part of achieving lasting weight loss and long-term happiness. It's important to remember that everyone's body is different, and a method that works for someone else might not be right for you.

Instead of comparing yourself to others or trying to meet an unrealistic ideal, try to accept and love your body for what it is. This positive attitude can help you make healthier choices and keep a balanced diet. When you start feeling good about your body, you focus less on the number on the scale and more on being strong, healthy, and confident.

One good way to start feeling better about your body is by practicing self-care and self-love. Be kind to yourself and do things that make you feel good, both physically and mentally. This might include regular exercise, getting plenty of sleep, and eating nutritious foods that nourish your body.

Another key part of feeling good about your body is to make sure you're around positive influences. Look for support from friends, family, or maybe a therapist who can help you develop a good relationship with food and how you see your body. Remember, losing weight in a lasting way isn't just about changing how your body looks; it's also about feeling better mentally and emotionally.

By accepting and loving your body image, you can take a healthier and more lasting approach to losing weight. Concentrate on loving and taking care of your body, and the other pieces will fall into place. When you treat your body with care and respect, you're more likely to find joy in the journey of staying healthy.

Chapter 10: Building Your Support System

When you start trying to lose weight, having people around to support you can really make a big difference. Being around people who understand and support what you're trying to do can keep you motivated and help you stick to your goals. In this chapter, we'll talk about why it's important to have a support system and how you can build one effectively.

Your support system can be made up of friends, family, coworkers, or even people you meet in online groups that focus on weight loss and healthy living. Look for people who will encourage you, say positive things, and listen to you when you need to talk. Having people to support you can also help you deal with any problems or setbacks that come up.

One way to create a support system is to be open about your goals and what you need from others. Tell them how they can help you, whether it's going for a walk together, making healthy meals together, or just checking in with you to see how you're doing. Surround yourself with people who believe in you and your ability to succeed and who will help you keep going.

Besides friends and family, think about getting help from a professional like a nutritionist or a personal trainer. They have expert knowledge and can give you advice that fits your personal needs. These experts can help you make a diet and exercise plan that's just for you, which can help you succeed over the long term.

Remember, losing weight and keeping it off isn't something you have to do alone. By having a strong group of supporters, you're more likely to achieve your goals and live healthily for many years. Fill your life with positive vibes and supportive people, and you'll see yourself changing and succeeding.

Importance of Social Support in Achieving Goals

In your quest for lasting weight loss, having a strong group of supporters is incredibly important. The value of having others to support you in achieving your goals is huge. Studies have shown that people who have friends, family, or even online groups backing them are more likely to be successful in losing weight.

When you have people who understand what you're trying to do and support you, they can help keep you motivated and accountable. They can celebrate your successes with you, give you advice, and be there for you when things get hard. Being around positive people can help keep you dedicated to your weight loss goals.

Social support has been shown to improve the adoption and adherence to physical activity, as it increases accountability and motivation for the behavior[65]. Your network can also boost motivation to exercise and maintain a healthy lifestyle, as individuals may feel more accountable and encouraged by their supportive network[66].

---

[65]https://www2.worc.ac.uk/gjseper/documents/SOCIAL_SUPPORT_AS_A_STAGE_SPECIF IC_CORRELATE_OF_PHYSICAL_ACTIVITY.pdf
[66]https://www.trainerize.me/articles/the-power-of-social-support-enhancing-exercise-and-healthy-living/

Your support network can also help you deal with any challenges that come up. Whether it's managing cravings, making time for exercise, or getting past weight loss plateaus, the people who support you can offer useful advice and strategies. This help can be crucial in keeping you on the right path toward your goals.

Having people support you can also make you feel more confident and believe more in your ability to reach your weight loss goals. Knowing that there are people who believe in you and are cheering for you can give you an extra boost to keep going, even when it's hard.

In the sustainable weight loss plan in this book, having a personalized diet plan is important, but it's not the only thing that matters. Understanding how important it is to have support from others shows that losing weight is about more than just food. It's also about the people around you and how they can help you succeed.

Remember, you don't have to do this alone—rely on your support network and see how much easier it is to achieve your weight loss goals with their encouragement and help.

Enlisting Support from Friends, Family, and Professionals

Starting a weight loss journey can be much easier and more successful with a strong support system around you. Friends, family, and professionals can offer encouragement, keep you accountable, and give you helpful advice to keep you moving toward your goals.

Friends and family can be especially supportive during your weight loss journey. If you tell them about your goals, they can help keep you accountable and motivated. They can cheer you on when you achieve something, celebrate your successes, and be there to listen when you feel down. Furthermore, including your loved ones in your weight loss journey can make it more fun and allow for activities you can do together, like working out or cooking healthy meals. This not only helps you stick to your goals but also strengthens your relationships.

Alongside the support from friends and family, getting help from professionals like nutritionists, personal trainers, and healthcare providers can be very useful. These experts can give you personalized advice and guidance tailored to your needs. They can help you figure out the best eating and exercise plans that suit you and offer ongoing support as you work towards your goals.

Also, participating in group exercise can provide companionship support, which has been shown to be the most beneficial type of social support for exercise behavior[67].

Remember, losing weight in a sustainable way isn't just about sticking to a strict diet or exercise plan—it's about making changes to your lifestyle that you can keep up over time. By getting support from friends, family, and professionals, you build a strong base for success. This support system will help you keep on track in the long run. Use all the resources available to you, and don't hesitate to ask for help when you need it. With the

---

[67]https://www2.worc.ac.uk/gjseper/documents/SOCIAL_SUPPORT_AS_A_STAGE_SPECIF IC_CORRELATE_OF_PHYSICAL_ACTIVITY.pdf

right support, you can reach your weight loss goals and build a healthier, happier future for yourself.

Creating a Supportive Environment for Success

Creating a Supportive Environment for Success is crucial if you want to achieve and maintain weight loss. In this subchapter, we'll discuss how important it is to have a supportive environment to help you stay focused on your weight loss goals.

The first step in creating a supportive environment is to surround yourself with positive influences. This could involve finding a workout buddy, joining a support group, or getting a coach or mentor. Having someone who holds you accountable and offers encouragement can greatly impact your success in losing weight.

Another key part of creating a supportive environment is making sure your living space supports your goals. This involves removing unhealthy temptations from your pantry and fridge and stocking up on nutritious foods instead. Keeping healthy snacks easily accessible will help you resist the urge to eat unhealthy junk food when you feel hungry or have a craving. This setup not only helps you stick to healthy eating habits but also reinforces your commitment to your weight loss journey every time you make a food choice.

Besides filling your kitchen with healthy foods, it's also important to have a regular meal schedule and stick to it. This helps prevent random snacking and overeating by making sure your body gets the right nutrients at the right times. Having a meal plan keeps you organized and focused on your weight loss goals, as it reduces the temptation to grab whatever is quickest and easiest, which often isn't the healthiest choice.

Moreover, creating a supportive environment also involves taking good care of your mental and emotional health. Engaging in self-care activities like meditation, journaling, or spending time outdoors can greatly lower stress and boost your overall mindset. When you feel less stressed and more at peace, it's easier to stay motivated and keep your focus on your weight loss journey.

By building a supportive environment that looks after your physical, emotional, and mental health, you set the stage for long-term success in reaching your weight loss goals. Remember, achieving sustainable weight loss is not only about the food you eat but also about creating a living environment that supports your overall well-being.

Chapter 11: Putting it All Together: Creating Your Personalized Plan

In Chapter 11 of "Healthy You, " we'll bring everything you've learned together to help you make your own personal plan for lasting success. This chapter is where everything starts to come together—you'll use all the information you've gathered from the book and adjust it to fit your specific needs and goals.

Creating a plan that's just for you is key to lasting weight loss because everyone is different. Your body and your life are unique to you. What helps one person lose weight might not work for another, and that's why diets that are the same for everyone often don't lead to permanent weight loss. By making a plan that suits your own likes, habits, and health needs, you'll find it much easier to follow over the long term.

In this chapter, we'll guide you step by step on how to create your own personalized plan. First, we'll help you figure out what your goals are. Then, we'll look at what you currently eat, work out how many calories and nutrients you need, and help you plan your meals and snacks. We'll also give you advice on how to stick to your plan, how to deal with any problems that come up, and how to make changes to your plan when you need to.

By the end of Chapter 11, you'll have a clear and specific plan that fits your personal needs and likes. With this customized approach, you'll be ready to achieve lasting weight loss and keep up your results over time. Let's begin and make a plan that really works for you!

Steps to Create Your Personalized Diet Plan

Creating a personalized diet plan is a crucial step toward achieving your health and fitness goals. By following a structured approach, you can tailor your nutrition to meet your specific needs and preferences. Below is a detailed guide outlining the essential steps to create your personalized diet plan:

Step 1: Define Your Goals

Defining your goals is the foundational step in creating a personalized diet plan. Whether you aim to lose weight, gain muscle, maintain your current weight, or simply eat more healthily, clarifying your objectives will shape your meal plan and guide your choices. Understanding what you want to achieve is essential for designing a diet plan that aligns with your desired outcomes.

Step 2: Examine Your Existing Diet

Take a critical look at your current eating habits to assess what you typically consume, including portion sizes, meal timing, and food choices. This evaluation provides a starting point for creating a meal plan that suits your lifestyle. Understanding your current diet patterns helps identify areas for improvement and make necessary adjustments to align with your goals.

Step 3: Work Out How Many Calories and What Nutrients You Need

Determining your daily caloric needs is crucial and depends on factors such as your goals, age, activity level, and metabolic rate. Online calculators and nutrition apps can assist in estimating your daily caloric requirements. Additionally, planning your macronutrient ratios, such as carbohydrates, protein, and fat, based on your goals is essential for a balanced diet. Adjust these ratios according to your specific objectives, such as increasing protein intake for muscle building.

Step 4: Plan Your Meals and Snacks

Designing a daily eating schedule that suits your lifestyle is key to creating a successful diet plan. Consider the number of meals and snacks you prefer and allocate your daily calories accordingly. Focus on selecting whole, nutrient-dense foods like fruits, vegetables, lean proteins, whole grains, and healthy fats. Avoid or limit processed foods, sugary beverages, and excessive sodium. Ensure that each meal provides a balance of macronutrients to support your health and fitness goals.

By following these steps and incorporating personalized elements into your diet plan, you can create a sustainable and effective approach to nutrition that aligns with your individual needs and preferences. Consistency, flexibility, and a focus on nutrient-rich foods are key components of a successful personalized diet plan.

How to Stick to Your Diet Plan

Sticking to a diet plan is essential for achieving your health and fitness goals. One strategy to facilitate this is to set achievable and realistic goals that match your lifestyle and preferences. Try not to aim for goals that are too ambitious, as they can lead to frustration. Making steady progress toward your goals is essential for long-term success and sticking to your plans.

It is best to create an eating plan that includes foods you like and offers a good mix of nutrients. Make sure to include lots of fruits, vegetables, whole grains, lean proteins, and nuts in your diet. These foods are not only good for you but are also satisfying, which makes it easier to stay committed to your food regime.

Moreover, instead of trying to change everything at once, make small, gradual changes to your eating habits. Changing one thing at a time helps you get used to new ways of eating and helps you build lasting habits. Keep healthy foods in your kitchen and plan to make nutritious meals at home.

Celebrate your progress to stay motivated. Give yourself a reward when you reach small goals, like losing a few pounds or consistently following your plan. It's important to recognize your successes and to be gentle with yourself if you encounter setbacks. Use any slip-ups as chances to learn and improve rather than reasons to give up on your diet.

Finally, use a food diary or an app to keep track of what you eat every day. Writing down what you eat and drink can help you stay aware of your eating choices and help you control your diet. Keeping track of your meals also lets you spot patterns, make necessary changes, and stay committed to your eating plan[68].

How to Deal with Problems and Make Changes to Your Diet Plan

Dealing with challenges and making adjustments to your diet plan is a normal part of the process. What you can do is be sure

---

[68] https://www.webmd.com/obesity/features/7-ways-get-your-diet-off-good-start

to regularly check how your diet plan is working and look for areas that might need some changes. Evaluate how well you're doing, what you like, and what results you're seeing to make sure your diet plan fits your current needs. Keeping your plan customized helps ensure it stays useful and effective for you.

Another great strategy is to keep learning about nutrition and healthy eating. Use a structured three-step approach: first, learn the basics; second, apply what you've learned to your eating habits; and third, adjust based on the results. This education is key to helping you make smart choices and tweaks to your diet plan.

Finally, try to keep your diet plan flexible to match any changes in your lifestyle, tastes, or goals. Avoid strict rules that can make you feel frustrated or deprived. Try to simplify your plan by focusing on whole, nutrient-rich foods and using straightforward strategies that are easy to stick to over time[69].

Summary of Core Concepts and Strategies

In this subchapter, we'll recap the main ideas and strategies from the book "Healthy You."

A major point we've talked about in the book is how important it is to have a diet plan that's made just for you if you want to successfully lose weight and keep it off. We understand that everyone is different, and there's no single diet plan that works for everyone. By making a diet plan that fits your own

---

[69]https://www.ideafit.com/personal-training/nutrition-adherence-making-lifestyle-changes-that-stick/

needs, likes, and way of life, you're much more likely to see long-lasting results.

Another important idea we talk about is the need to eat fewer calories than your body uses to lose weight, which is called creating a calorie deficit. However, it's very important not to cut your calories too much because this can be bad for your health and make it hard to keep the weight off in the long run.

We also explain why it's crucial to eat a variety of nutrient-rich foods. This includes fruits, vegetables, whole grains, lean proteins, and healthy fats. By eating whole, unprocessed foods, you provide your body with the essential nutrients it needs to function well and support your weight loss efforts. This approach not only helps in shedding pounds but also enhances your overall health.

We also share tips for dealing with common problems that can make it hard to lose weight and maintain good weight. These include emotional eating, feeling unmotivated, and dealing with social pressures. By facing these issues directly and learning healthy ways to cope with them, you can move forward in your weight loss journey feeling strong and capable.

The main ideas and strategies we talk about in this book are meant to help you take charge of your health, lose weight in a way that you can maintain, and come up with a diet plan that fits your individual needs. With commitment, patience, and the right guidance, you can change your lifestyle for the better and reach your weight loss goals.

Call to Action and Encouragement for Readers to Take Action

In this final subchapter, I want to encourage everyone who has read "Healthy You" to take a big step forward. It's time to really focus on your health and commit to achieving long-lasting success in your journey to lose weight.

I urge all of you to start making changes today. Don't wait for the perfect time or the ideal situation to begin. Start right now by taking small, easy steps that you can handle. These small steps will lead to major changes over time. It could be something as simple as stopping drinking sugary beverages, adding more vegetables to your diet, or making a plan to exercise regularly. Every small action you take adds up and makes a difference.

Remember, lasting weight loss isn't about quick fixes or crash diets. It's about making changes to your lifestyle that will improve your health and well-being for many years. By using the personalized diet plans provided in this book, you already have what you need to be successful.

I want to remind you that you can reach your weight loss goals. Believe in yourself and your ability to change your habits for the better. Make sure you have supportive friends and family around you who will cheer you on. And remember to be kind to yourself during this process.

So, I'm challenging you to start today. Make a promise to yourself and your health. Begin using the diet plans from this book and watch as you start to lose weight. You have the ability to change your life for the better—now is the time to do it. Good luck on your journey to lasting weight loss!

Chapter 12: Conclusion: Embracing Your Journey

Congratulations on finishing the book "Healthy You." You've learned a lot about how having a diet plan that fits your personal needs is key to losing weight and keeping it off for good. Now, it's time to keep going and move forward on your path to a healthier and happier life.

Think about what you've learned from this book. Remember, losing weight the right way isn't about quick fixes or the same solution for everyone. It takes real commitment, patience, and a readiness to change your lifestyle permanently. By creating a diet plan that fits just right for you, you're laying down the groundwork for lasting success.

Keep using what you've learned here and build on it. Every step you take is a step toward a better you. Good luck as you continue your journey to sustainable weight loss!

Make sure to celebrate your progress, no matter how small it might seem. Every little step you take toward a healthier lifestyle is important and moves you in the right direction. It's normal to face setbacks along the way, but don't let them stop you. Instead, see these challenges as chances to learn and become stronger.

As you keep moving forward with your weight loss goals, it's helpful to be around supportive people like friends, family, or others who are also focused on health. Talk about your successes, the challenges you face, and what you hope to achieve with people who support and motivate you. This community can be a big help in keeping you on track.

In conclusion, your journey to lasting weight loss is a very personal and empowering experience. When you make a diet plan that fits just right for you, stay dedicated to your goals, and get help and encouragement from others, you're really setting yourself up for long-term success. Remember, this isn't just about losing weight—it's about leading a healthier, happier, and more fulfilling life. Embrace your journey, and look forward to the amazing changes that are coming your way.

Reflection on the Journey and Encouragement for Continued Growth

In this final subchapter, let's take a moment to think about the journey you've been on toward lasting weight loss. It's been full of highs and lows, challenges and victories, and most importantly, it has been a journey of personal growth and discovery. As you look back at how much you've achieved, make sure to celebrate every bit of progress and every success, no matter how small they might seem.

However, your journey doesn't stop here. Keeping the weight off is a commitment for life, and it's important to keep taking care of both your body and mind as you go forward. Remember, everyone's journey is different, and what helps one person might not help another. It's crucial to listen to your body, notice how different foods affect you, and change your diet and lifestyle as needed.

As you keep moving toward your long-term goals, it's important to be patient and kind to yourself. Remember, Rome wasn't built in a day. Achieving lasting weight loss requires time and commitment. Don't get upset by setbacks or times when your progress seems to stall; instead, see these moments as chances to learn and improve. It's also helpful to be part of a community of supportive people who share your goals and can encourage and motivate you along the way.

Most importantly, believe in your ability to reach your weight loss goals and lead a healthier, happier life. Believe in yourself, keep your eyes on your goals, and don't give up. With commitment, persistence, and a diet plan tailored to your needs, achieving sustainable weight loss is definitely possible. Enjoy the journey, celebrate every success, and keep working towards a healthier, happier you.